Working with People with Learning Disabilities

Working with People with Learning Disabilities

Systemic Approaches

EDITED BY VICTORIA JONES AND

MARK HAYDON-LAURELUT

BLOOMSBURY ACADEMIC

LONDON · NEW YORK · OXFORD · NEW DELHI · SYDNEY

BLOOMSBURY ACADEMIC
Bloomsbury Publishing Plc
50 Bedford Square, London, WC1B 3DP, UK
1385 Broadway, New York, NY 10018, USA
29 Earlsfort Terrace, Dublin 2, Ireland

BLOOMSBURY, BLOOMSBURY ACADEMIC and the Diana logo
are trademarks of Bloomsbury Publishing Plc

First published in 2019 by RED GLOBE PRESS
Reprinted by Bloomsbury Academic, 2022, 2023

A catalogue record for this book is available from the British Library.

A catalogue record for this book available from the Library of Congress.

ISBN: PB: 978-1-3520-0536-3
ePDF: 978-1-3520-0537-0
ePub: 978-1-3503-1070-4

Printed and bound in Great Britain

To find out more about our authors and books visit
www.bloomsbury.com and sign up for our newsletters.

Nora Bateson

'It is within our interactions that entirely unanticipated possibilities are found.'

Contents

List of Figures

List of Tables

List of Reflective Practice Boxes

These boxes are designed to offer questions and exercises that enhance reflective and reflexive practice. You may choose to use them individually, to initiate team discussions, or in training situations.

Acknowledgements

To Seren, Darrah and Hester for their support, encouragement and just being generally awesome; and The Family Institute in Wales who invited Victoria into the joys of thinking systemically.

To wonderful Corinne and Etienne who kept things (Mark) afloat while editing this book; to the Kensington Consultation Centre, the Houston Galveston Institute and Taos Institute who taught me so much; and to the many others (some, but not all, of whom are authors in this text) who have shared their systemic approaches.

And to Karl Nunkoosing our teacher, mentor and friend and the many people with learning disabilities and their families who have taught us so much.

List of Contributors

Dr Sandra Baum is Head of Learning Disabilities Psychological Services for Oxleas NHS Foundation Trust. She is a consultant clinical psychologist, systemic psychotherapist and an honorary senior lecturer at UCL. Sandra has worked with people with learning disabilities for over 30 years.

Darren Bleek is a clinical team manager and systemic practitioner currently living in South Devon, UK. He works in the Intensive Assessment Treatment Team West (Devon), a multidisciplinary team supporting people with a learning disability who are experiencing distress. The 'Guide to a Good Day' is one of the tools this team may use as part of its work with individuals.

Dr Sarah Brown is a clinical psychologist working with children and families in Gwent, and children in specialist education in England. She has an interest in community psychology, holding social justice and empowerment of families and communities as central to her practice.

Samuel Coe is a senior assistant psychologist working part time at an Assessment and Treatment Unit and also in a community team for people with learning disabilities. He is soon to become the learning disabilities team business manager. He enjoys playing sports, including football, cricket and squash, and can often be found looking for bargains in charity shops.

Dr Sarah Coles is a clinical psychologist, supervisor, and systemic psychotherapist. She worked for 8 years with adults with learning disabilities in Oxfordshire as part of a multidisciplinary team; teaches on a number of doctoral courses in clinical psychology (both systemic and learning disabilities modules); and works as a family therapist with children and adolescents in a CAMH (Child and Adolescent Mental Health) service in Oxfordshire. She likes reading and yoga.

Leanne Coleman is a proud mother of two. She is an advocate for children with learning difficulties and has a specific interest in children's rights. She loves the outdoors and inspiring quotes!

Dr Helen Ellis-Caird is a principal lecturer at the University of Hertfordshire and a clinical psychologist working with people with learning disabilities. She is a member of the British Psychological Society Ethics Committee and cares deeply about the ethics of clinical practice. Her favourite times are swimming in the sea and playing on the beach with her family and friends.

Dr Karin Fuchs works as a consultant clinical psychologist in services for people with learning disabilities in West Sussex (Sussex Partnership NHS Trust). Before that, since qualifying, she worked in South London and East London. She has always had an interest in applying systemic ideas and ways of working to her work with people with learning disabilities, staff teams and networks of concern. She is also interested in integrating systemic approaches into supporting people presenting with behaviour that challenges, and has developed and led enhanced support provision in both Southwark and West Sussex.

Dr Amy Hamilton-Roberts is a qualified educational psychologist, practising as a psychologist for Newport City Council and as a professional tutor on the Doctorate in Educational Psychology at Cardiff University. Amy describes herself as a humanistic psychologist who strongly believes in inclusivity.

Dr Cathy Harding has worked for the past 15 years as a clinical psychologist in community, inpatient and supported living services, primarily within South Wales and always within multidisciplinary teams. She actively seeks to ensure that people's histories are integrated into their care and that individuals feel empowered within their lives; she also enjoys baking and eating cake!

Dr Mark Haydon-Laurelut, Editor is a systemic psychotherapist and senior lecturer in the Department of Psychology at the University of Portsmouth. His therapeutic work is primarily with adults with learning disabilities and their systems of significant relationships. He enjoys making music and anything to do with the sea.

Dr Caley Hill has been alongside people who have a learning disability throughout her adult life. Her experience of exploring stories and context with the intention of increasing control and choice for people has been overwhelmingly positive and sustaining. She currently works as a clinical psychologist in the NHS, based in South Wales.

Victoria Jones, Editor is a specialist systemic family psychotherapist, a registered nurse for people with learning disabilities and a Senior Fellow of the Higher Education Academy. She is a feminist and loves purple (which for her represents power, understanding, respect, pride, love and elegance).

Katarina Luce is the mother of three children, one of whom has complex needs. She co-founded SENDawelcome to instigate local change for children with disabilities, their families and the wider community. She is totally committed to thinking a great deal about doing more exercise.

Dr Henrik Lynggaard is a clinical psychologist and systemic psychotherapist who has worked in the field of learning disabilities for more than 20 years. He has published widely and, along with Sandra Baum, is the co-editor of *Intellectual Disabilities: A Systemic Approach* (Karnac, 2006).

Abby Maitland is a family and systemic psychotherapist and a registered social worker. Having worked within CAMHS LD (Child and Adolescent Mental Health Learning Disability Services) for many years, she is currently Operational Manager for Specialist CAMHS. Abby is a strong advocate for empowering marginalised voices. She enjoys long walks with her partner and their two dogs.

Dr Jennifer McElwee is a clinical psychologist who enjoys thinking creatively about making connections with people who communicate in ways other than language. She is passionate about promoting and developing inclusive communities.

Dr Karl Nunkoosing has been engaged in the lives of people who experience learning difficulties, and their supporters, for over 50 years: 'Yes, I am old; alas, without the wisdom that comes with age. So I am still learning, often from the lives of people on the margins, so that I can do my job as a principal lecturer at the Department of Psychology, University of Portsmouth.'

Dr Lloyd Purdy is a general practitioner and systemic family therapist currently living and working in Vancouver, Canada. He previously worked as a part of the South Hams and West Devon Learning Disabilities Team together with Darren Bleek at a time when the 'Guide to a Good Day' was being developed.

Dr Bethan Ramsey is a clinical psychologist working in London with people with learning disabilities and their communities. She draws on systemic and narrative ideas and practices, and loves sharing these ideas with others and learning from those she works with.

Dr Peggy Ravoux is a clinical psychologist and the lead for the Southwark Enhanced Intervention Service (South London and Maudsley NHS Trust). As a PBS (positive behaviour support) and systemic practitioner, she is passionate about supporting clients with learning disabilities with behaviours that challenge, and their families. She is interested in creative arts and thinking 'outside the box'.

Dr Donna Reeve is a disabled academic in disability studies who is best known for her research and writing about psycho-emotional disablism. She has an ongoing interest in the experiences of disabled clients in therapy and in her spare time makes jewellery.

Selma Rikberg Smyly worked for many years as a consultant clinical psychologist and systemic practitioner in a multidisciplinary NHS team in Oxford. She currently works freelance as a trainer and supervisor for psychologists working systemically in services for people with learning disabilities. She recently became a grandmother and is greatly enjoying her new status!

Dr Lorna Robbins is a systemic family therapist and consultant clinical psychologist specialising in working with people with learning disabilities (LD). She is the Clinical Lead for LD Psychology, and also Team Manager for the Specialist Health Team (LD) in Somerset. Lorna loves living by the coast, and her favourite times are walks with family and friends, with stops for tea and cakes.

Dr Ian Smillie is a qualified educational psychologist who divides his working week between practising as a psychologist and service manager for the 'Parents Plus' (parenting) service at Cardiff Flying Start, and working as a professional tutor on the Doctorate in Educational Psychology at Cardiff University. He describes himself as a humanist, a cyclist, and a gardener (but is often too tired for much of the latter).

Dr Julie Steel is a clinical psychologist and systemic practitioner. She works in an adult learning disability team three days a week, and for the other two is a clinical and academic tutor at Salomons. She is vegan, loves dogs and likes swimming in lakes.

Jane Steeples is a specialist counsellor with experience of working as a carer, and a therapist with adults with learning disabilities, parent carers and staff teams. She has particular interest in attachment- and trauma-focused work; she likes playing badminton and has a house rabbit called Molly.

Dr Julia Young is an educational psychologist currently working in Early Years and with schools in a local authority in the UK. She is interested in how systemic approaches can benefit vulnerable children, families and education professionals; she loves learning and being outdoors.

Dr Esther Wilcox is a consultant clinical psychologist. Since qualifying she has worked with adults with learning disabilities and currently works in an NHS specialist hospital. She is interested in systemic ideologies and the impact of current constructions of 'truth'. Esther loves spending time with family and friends, reading and her local parkrun.

Introduction

Victoria Jones and Mark Haydon-Laurelut

This book is written for everyone who stands in solidarity with people who have been labelled with a learning disability. We hope that people who themselves live with the label and its effects, their families, friends and those who seek to support them in any capacity (e.g. as educator, health professional, social worker, personal assistant, or therapist) will each find something in this text that speaks to them and offers practical ideas and resources. Solidarity is inherently an active position to take. It is not possible to stand alongside someone who is systematically devalued by society to the extent that their very existence and right to life is challenged, for example through antenatal screening and termination or premature death through poor health outcomes (e.g. Heslop et al., 2013), and not be moved to make change happen. Whilst it is a truism that the only person anyone has the power to really change is themselves and that, as a consequence of this, shifts in our lives and communities must *start* with us, systemic approaches show us that we are also all part of an interconnected web. Thinking systemically, it is possible for us and the changes that we *can* make to be the 'difference that makes a difference' (Bateson, 1972, p. 465). Systemic ideas offer us hope that we have the ability to effect positive change.

After many years of experience alongside people labelled with learning disabilities and as a consequence of our individual journeys towards becoming systemic family psychotherapists, it strikes us that the process of making the right conversation with the right people in the right place at the right time can often be enough to effect a change that can both make a difference and create new possibilities. Our challenge is to know *who* the right people are and *how* to actively engage them *and ourselves* in a different kind of 'conversation'. We consider that the body of work regarding family systems theory and its application offers numerous useful resources for those seeking to join with people with learning disabilities in their pursuit of a good life.

With such a diverse potential audience we have been challenged more than ever to be conscious of the language that we use. Consideration of language is also an inherently systemic concern, recognising that 'we construct our realities in conversations and relationships with others and that these realities are constituted through language' Fredman (2006, p. 8). Words become meaningful when we use them in relationships and contexts. This makes it necessary for us to ensure that we coordinate with others in the systems that we are trying to change to manage what we mean by the words we use, how we are using them and the pragmatic effect that they may have on others (Pearce & Cronen, 1980).

'Learning disability' is a current legislative term in the United Kingdom that is applied to an extremely diverse group of women, men and children. This label is enough to make it possible for 'us' to edit a book that 'you' will read about 'them'. Yet the only thing that this heterogeneous group of individuals specifically have in common is that early in their life a 'professional person' (someone afforded power on the basis of their 'knowledge', skills and role) identified that they had some difficulty understanding new concepts, communicating ideas and managing socially (Department of Health, 2001). Learning disability is a socially constructed term – this is evidenced by the differences in whom the label is applied to, across time, culture, geographical context and profession (Baum and Lyngaard, 2006) and by the range of labels that are utilised, for example special educational needs (in educational contexts); intellectual impairment (Australasia); and intellectual disability (US). Terms officially change when people in power (ultimately governments) decide that they will. However, the term 'learning disability' was in popular use in the UK long before Stephen Dorrell, the incumbent health minister, announced in 1992 that henceforth policy would make use of that particular label. Indeed, it is only in this decade that the campaign for 'Rosa's Law' has been enacted in the US, finally consigning the much-derided term 'mental retardation' to the history books.

This constitutes a 'discourse of domination' (Freire, 1972). When we ignore the language preferred by self-advocates themselves, we use a position of power to control their language and meaning-making, in this case in something as significant as how people are labelled, identified and, ultimately, perceived by themselves and others. If we are to act ethically and attend to the rights of those with least power, we have a duty to consider the terms that they choose to use. For example, a group of self-advocates representing organisations of people with learning disabilities from across South Wales agreed that their preferred term, if people *had* to have a label, was *people with learning disabilities*. However, other self-advocates in England have clearly stated their preference for the term *people with learning difficulties*. The first group prioritises legislative terms and common language whilst the second group makes the social model of disability its highest context marker. This is a great example of how *theoretical approach* and *context* impact upon the appropriateness of any term and why we should always be curious and collaborative about our use of terms and language.

Recognising that each contributor to this text works in different professional and community contexts, we decided not to specify the terminology that people should use throughout the book. This was a deliberate decision not to buy in to thinking that we know better about individuals, their theories or their contexts than anyone else. To some extent we have declined to join a discourse of domination and have invited authors to consider the terms that they have chosen to use. That said, we have suggested that authors are cautious with the term *intellectual disability* which, whilst increasingly in use in Australasia, Canada, Éire, academia and psychology, is not a term we have ever heard someone use to refer to themselves.

We have also sought to amplify the voices of people labelled with learning disabilities themselves in the discourse generated in this book. Across the United Kingdom, Northern Ireland and the Republic of Ireland current legislation and guidance in health and social care endorses a culture of co-production, partnership, inclusion and involvement (Northern Ireland Assembly, 2009; Department of Health, 2014; National Advocacy Unit et al., 2014; Welsh Government, 2014; Scottish Government, 2017). Each contributor to this text was invited to write collaboratively and incorporate the voices of people with learning disabilities and their families into their chapter; the majority met with challenges. Whilst we are guided to work in partnership, the organisations and professional systems in which we work are rarely equipped to support, enable or permit us to do so. For example, jointly writing a chapter with someone who is considered a 'client' risks breaking policies on confidentiality and professional ethics. All materials presented in this book have received relevant consents and material has been anonymised where appropriate. However, if we are to truly work in partnership with people who use services then shifts in our thinking about control and ownership are required. We need to find ways to challenge the paternalistic and protective stances of the powerful services that currently threaten to undermine collaboration and creativity.

Reflective practice is a key element of training in a wide range of professional programmes (Dallos & Stedmon, 2009). Therapeutic traditions also emphasise reflexive thinking to promote best practice and professional development. This entails discovering our own core values and ways of making sense of things and considering the effect they may have had on our actions. Burnham (1993) provided a structure for approaching systemic reflexivity when he distinguished between *why* something is done (approach), the *context* in which it happens (method) and *what it is* that happens (technique).

> Approach relates to those personal prejudices, aesthetic preferences and theoretical concepts shaping the social construction of training cultures, team discourse and supervisory relationships. ... Method relates to the organisational patterns used both to set forth and bring forth the approach. ... Technique relates to those specific supervisory practices that can be observed and even 'counted' by an observer of the activity.
>
> (Burnham, 1993, p. 351)

How this book is organised

This book is organised using Burnham's Approach, Method, Technique structure (1992). The first section contains chapters that introduce you to key theories and concepts that are critical considerations when exploring systemic practice with people with learning disabilities and consider the questions: what is a systemic approach? What does 'learning disability' really mean? How are models of disability relevant? How are stories important? And how do I work systemically with referrals?

The second section of the book considers systemic ideas in specific contexts that are common for people labelled with learning disability: family life; education; community teams; crisis intervention services; and assessment and treatment units. This section also includes the application of systemic thinking during periods of transition such as in palliative care and bereavement; recovery in mental health; diagnoses and supervision. The final chapter in this section, Chapter 15, considers the context of research, evidence-based practice and practice-based evidence.

The third section is designed as a reference toolkit of ideas and techniques that you can try and adopt as you expand your systemic thinking and practice: prejudices; reflecting conversations including a model for after restraint; roles and positions; models used in Coordinated Management of Meaning; reframing; curiosity; cultural genograms; both/and; irreverence; engaging people; relational reflexivity; and the Social Graces acronym to help develop reflexivity regarding diversity.

If after all this you would like to find out more about systemic approaches and professional development opportunities, including training as a systemic practitioner or family therapist, we have added a signpost to relevant organisations. It is probably fair to say that systemic theorists are not renowned for their use of plain English so we have also incorporated a glossary of key terms.

How you will read and interpret this book will vary according to a wide range of factors including your culture, experience, age and educational background. Systemic thinkers place great emphasis on reflection and reflexively considering your own context, background and ideas and how they may influence you and others. For this reason you will find that many of chapters are written in the first person and authors have taken time to articulate their background and professional role to help you consider their position or stance. Chapter 10 in Section 2, by Hill and Harding, recognising that we make new meaning in relationship and language, is presented as a reflective and reflexive conversation between the authors.

In collating the chapters we have tried to bear witness to the range of services and ideas that exist. Some are leading edge whilst others are trying new ways to address service deficiencies and old challenges. We have deliberately included ideas that stretch our comfort zones to moderate the limits that our prejudices and biases may impose on the discourse (or conversation of thoughts and ideas) presented in this book. The chief criterion for inclusion was a desire to share creative ways of incorporating aspects of systemic thinking into our practice with people who have been labelled with learning disabilities and the systems around them. We think that these ideas can offer a myriad of opportunities to make a difference and effect positive change.

It is important to acknowledge the paradox inherent in the production of a book such as this: we have utilised our privileged access to power and knowledge to create a discourse around a group of people whom we have named as 'other' (or at least in some way like each other and different to us). In so doing we may have employed our own personal, academic and professional goals to make a difference. If this book is well received, it may even further assert that position of power and knowledge. However, whilst virtually all systemic books and the majority of those published about people with learning disabilities are in a format that excludes them, we have sought to ensure each chapter starts with a summary that *with good support* might be more accessible to anyone who is interested to find out more about how to use systemic ideas in a context that includes people labelled with learning disabilities. We encourage you to find ways to share the ideas in this book with the individuals you serve as well as with those who work alongside or employ you.

In editing this book we have had to reflectively, reflexively and recursively consider everything we think we know individually and collectively (Andersen, 1995). Looking through a systemic lens has brought about a reframing and greater awareness of our practice, knowledge, beliefs and prejudices in relation to women, men and children labelled with learning disability. We hope that the ideas in this book will offer similar insights, challenges and opportunities to you.

References

Andersen, T. (1995). *Reflecting Processes: Acts of Informing and Forming in the Reflecting Team in Action Collaborative Processes in Family Therapy* (pp. 11–37). New York: The Guildford Press.

Bateson, G. (1972). *Steps to an Ecology of Mind*. Chicago, IL: Chandler Publications.

Baum, S. & Lyngaard, H. (2006). *Intellectual Disabilities: A Systemic Approach*. London: Karnac.

Burnham, J. (1992). Approach – Method – Technique: Making distinctions and creating connections. *Human Systems: The Journal of Systemic Consultation & Management*, 3, 3–26.

Burnham, J. (1993). Systemic supervision: The evolution of reflexivity in the context of the supervisory relationship. *Human Systems*, 4, 349–381.

Dallos, R. & Stedmon, J. (2009). Flying over the swampy lowlands: Reflective and reflexive Practice. In R. Dallos & J. Stedmon (eds), *Reflective Practice in Psychotherapy and Counselling* (pp. 1–22). Milton Keynes: Open University Press.

Department of Health. (2001). *Valuing People: A New Strategy for Learning Disability for the 21st Century.* London: Department of Health.

Department of Health. (2014). *The Care Act.* London: Her Majesty's Stationery Office.

Fredman, G. (2006). Working systemically with intellectual disability: Why not? In S. Baum, and H. Lyngaard, *Intellectual Disabilities: A Systemic Approach.* London: Karnac.

Freire, P. (1972). *Pedagogy of the Oppressed.* New York: Penguin.

Heslop, P., Blair, P., Fleming, P., Hoghton, M., Marriott, A. & Russ, L. (2013). *Confidential Inquiry into Premature Deaths of People with Learning Disabilities (CIPOLD): Final Report.* Bristol: Norah Fry Research Centre.

National Advocacy Unit, Health Service Executive in Partnership with the National Disability Unit, and the National Disability Authority (2014). *National Guidelines on Accessible Health and Social Care Services – a Guidance Document for Staff on the Provision of Accessible Services for All.* www.hse.ie/eng/services/yourhealthservice/access/natguideaccessibleservices/natguideaccessibleservices.pdf (accessed 25 February 2018).

Northern Ireland Assembly. (2009). *Health and Social Care (Reform) Act (Northern Ireland).* United Kingdom: UK Stationery Office.

Pearce, W. B. & Cronen, V. E. (1980). *Communication, Action, and Meaning: The Creation of Social Realities.* New York: Praeger.

Scottish Government. (2017). *Health and Social Care Standards My Support, My Life.* Edinburgh: Scottish Government.

Welsh Government. (2014). *The Social Services and Well Being (Wales) Act.* Cardiff: Welsh Government.

Section I

Introduction

Section 1 addresses the level of 'Approach' (Burnham, 1992). This level considers the theoretical ideas and concepts that influence and inspire what we do and how we do it. However, it also expands much further than our ways of knowing things, by incorporating all the values, beliefs, prejudices and assumptions that guide us in selecting the theories and concepts that influence both our practice and our orientation towards it. Indeed, it includes the very factors that inspire us to be allied with people labelled with learning disabilities. Each of us will have different elements that contribute to our approach. Equally, each profession, service, organisation and team will draw on a more, or less, identifiable range of concepts, ideas, principles, values and theories that influence how they decide and enact who they work with, what they do and how they do it.

We consider there are some key approaches that are fundamental considerations for all people who wish to be allies to women, men and children who have been labelled with learning disabilities. Firstly, we offer the concept that we all make sense of our existence in relationship and communication with other people, that is, in systems or systemically. Following this introduction to the systemic approach we also include a consideration of the way that the term 'learning disability' itself is socially constructed; an exploration of the ways that we consider and understand disabling barriers; an examination of how we make sense of our world using narrative ideas; and, for people trying to apply these ideas in their practice, a review of how to begin to work systemically with referrals. This is an introduction to fundamental approaches. We fully expect that each person's list will be much bigger and broader, and we invite you to consider all the ideologies, theories, beliefs and ways of knowing things that influence your thinking, writing and actions.

Reference

Burnham, J. (1992). Approach – Method – Technique: Making distinctions and creating connections. *Human Systems: the Journal of Systemic Consultation & Management,* 3, 3–26.

1

What is a Systemic Approach?

Mark Haydon-Laurelut and Victoria Jones

Accessible summary

- A systemic approach is interested in what happens between people.

- We are interested in how people and ideas come together.

- We are always connected in many ways to the world.

- Systemic thinking and systemic therapy and practice have changed over decades and collaborating with people has become important.

Woven together

> *woven together*
> *lives connected by stories*
> *We stand stronger now*

> Karen Holford (2017, p. 80)

A systemic approach foregrounds our connected world. We live our lives in systems: systems of language (Anderson & Goolishian, 1988), the systems of our physical bodies, the myriad social contexts in which we come to be ourselves – economic, political, our families – and the institutions in which we live and work. All these contexts, and more, inform who we are and how we make sense of the world. As Holford notes, we are 'woven together'. We are a *'richness that cannot be undone'* (Bateson, 2016, p. 27, our emphasis). And yet some of the ways in which we understand the world fail to reflect this richness, pass over the way in which we are woven together and, we suggest, leave untapped the strength of our connections. A systemic approach emphasises each person's rich and unique complexity, reminding us that we can never fully understand anyone, and that everyone deserves to be recognised as a person who is always developing and cannot be neatly summed up in a label, diagnosis, clinical description or formulation. Systemic approaches (in common with person-centred approaches (see, for example, Lay & Kirk, 2014)) seek rich stories of unique individuals and their network of relationships. We might look inside ourselves to discover 'who we are' and yet a systemic view cautions against this as the only manner in which we might understand the self:

> Identity is the result of countless conversations entertained with significant people. The conversation becomes restricted when the illusion appears that identity is autonomous, and exists independently and a-historically from the context of which it is a part. In that case a person becomes obsessed with 'who am I' and 'who are you' questions, which all too often result in a battle over whose description is correct.
>
> (Cecchin et al., 2010, p. 19)

Let us consider further what we mean by 'systemic'.

Relational

As professionals employed in evidence-based, outcome-driven, under-resourced services we might often find ourselves looking for problems or anomalies, what has caused them and how they are to be corrected. This is one possible way of thinking, one possible kind of practice. Systemic theorists, researchers and practitioners have shown over decades that this linear, problem-focused manner of understanding the world has its limitations and may itself be a cause of further problems. For example when we receive an invitation to work with a person it may describe someone, or some idea, or even some relationship as a 'cause' of the difficulties with which help is required. Systemic approaches allow us to view each named 'cause' as a punctuation or merely as one observer pointing to one part of the complex world and saying '*This is where it starts*!' For example, one partner, 'Ade', may be viewed as 'distant' from the other. Partner 'Ben' may be viewed as 'pursuing' the other. Both partners see the other's behaviour as the starting point for the unwanted pattern. 'If Ade did not withdraw so much I would not need to pursue him.' 'If Ben did not pursue as much I would not need to withdraw.' We might focus on the individual history of Ade and Ben, we might view Ade or Ben as more blameworthy and seek to alter their behaviour; however, a systemic circular and relational understanding draws our attention (and that of the partners) to the pattern of withdraw-pursue-withdraw-pursue and so on (we could have begun that pattern at any point). By focusing on the pattern rather than an individual we seek to reduce the constraining effects of blame on the partners. As we begin to work with individuals, couples, families and organisations we find that at the heart of many difficulties and conflicts are differences in punctuation, or the when, where, who and what was considered the cause of a problem. The systemic concept of feedback is crucial here. People often do not react in predictable ways to the communications of others. Unlike in the medical model where an infection causes an inflammation (Watzlawick et al., 1997, cited in Hedges, 2005) or a fall causes a bruise, communications occur in multiple contexts and can be understood in multiple ways. This can make it difficult to be sure of the effect of a particular communication and, as we have seen above in the example of Ade and Ben, cause and effect may have a circular and more complex relationship (see Hedges, 2005, p. 14). This kind of circular, relational thinking can help us to make sense of and reconfigure patterns. Consider Murray's (2005) description of a circular pattern below. Murray is describing the ways in which some people with a label of severe learning disability may be seen as not possessing an internal psychological reality. Murray describes this as the denial of psychological reality. Murray hypothesises a circular pattern in the form of a vicious circle. By doing so she is able to show how this pattern may be exited:

> We only begin to attend, in any meaningful sense of the word, to another's well-being when we acknowledge the reality of their internal experience. Such attention in turn elicits richer and more complete pictures of that internal reality. Just as the absence of empathy and absence of respect operate as cause and effect of one another in a vicious circle of exclusion; so does their presence, working in mirror image of the same dynamic, create the virtuous circle of inclusion.
>
> (Murray, 2005, pp. 40–41)

This example highlights how ideas as well as people are also in relation to each other. In taking a respectful position we encourage connection with the psychological reality of the person, in turn encouraging further respect and so on.

Box 1.1 Reflective questions on the ideas I favour

What ideas in your practice would you like to cultivate?

What other ideas and practices would these ideas encourage?

Appreciation

When a family or organisation finds themselves in difficulty and cannot find a way of going on we can, through a systemic approach, seek to understand the patterns of interaction between members of that family or organisation, the ways in which people talk, what they notice, the stories they tell, the ways in which they listen, how they habitually interpret one another and what this creates. However, our questions cannot be neutral in their language or focus. We could always have used another word, always asked another question. One response to this is to consider working appreciatively (Cooperrider & Srivastva, 1987). When we work appreciatively we focus our questions on asking about abilities, strengths, moments when the problems were less apparent and what it is people intend and value. How is it that people have achieved what they have? With whom have they done this? What might this say about them and their relationships? The ways in which we ask questions are powerful and in asking appreciative questions we can support different kinds of conversation about the patterns of talking and being together people most value, and would be most interested in developing. Lang and McAdam write about the power of our questions:

> When we ask questions of people as they answer, emotions, relationships and the like are invoked in the living flow of experience. Thus through questioning you experience life. In the process of describing an event you potentially experience the event differently. Thus the stories we tell may begin to change or the potential is established for the event itself to take on a new meaning and significance ... As these changes of experience take place, relationships change and patterns of the way people act with each other, change.
>
> (Lang and McAdam, 2001, p. 17)

Box 1.2 Reflecting on questions

Think about the kinds of questions you ask:

What might be the effect on clients and families of the questions you ask during assessment?

What kinds of stories of identity, family life, of past and future do your questions help develop?

In what ways do the questions you ask in your workplace encourage stories of abilities and stories of deficit?

Collaboration and humility

[Gregory Bateson] saw ecological destruction as being caused by human linear-conscious purposefulness and by our conviction that we are somehow separate from the rest of the living world.

(Charlton, 2008, p. 5)

Recognising the ways in which we perceive, make sense of and act into the world entails a reflexive self-awareness (Pearce, 2011). This is the act of noticing how we notice. This noticing speaks to a central tenet of systemic approaches, that we do not take (in fact we do not consider it is possible to take) an objective observer position on the world. We are a part of the world and we cannot step out of it to view it. This is part of what it means to be 'woven' together. How we view our lives, our professional positions, those we support and those who support us always occurs in relation to multiple contexts including contexts of difference and power such as, but not limited to, disability, race, religion, gender and class (to find out about others see 'Diversity IS GRACE', Chapter 20). This awareness of the provisional nature of knowledge encourages a systemic humility. Whatever it is we know, there is more to it than this. In a book such as this you will find phrases such as '*I wonder*', '*How might we...*', '*I was curious about*', reflecting a humility of approach as practitioners engage in a 'shared inquiry' (Anderson, 1997) with their clients, or you, the reader, about their lives. The history of systemic thinking and practice can be broadly characterised as a movement from expert objective knower through to collaborative partner. When we work systemically what emerges is not as a result of a professional or client acting alone; our work is one of co-construction. This relationship to our work implies professional responsibility and influence but not control. If important people in a system are left out of the conversations (consider, for example, a behaviour support plan written without the participation of the person with a learning disability to whom it applies) we may miss important aspects of the persons life. Systemic practice concerns facilitating useful conversations that make a difference for (and between) those who consult with us.

Let us now consider how systemic thinking emerged.

The emergence of a field

Although forms of systems thinking have been present for millennia – for example Heraclitus and his notion that one cannot step into the same river twice (it is flowing and so are you) – systemic thinking and practice as an identifiable movement emerged over 60 years ago, with much development occurring in the Macy conferences beginning in the 1940s. These were meetings across disciplinary boundaries with anthropologists, psychologists, engineers, computer scientists and biologists, to name a few. The emerging fields of systems thinking and cybernetics (the science of information flow, control and communication) were not the property of one discipline, nor did they fit neatly into anyone university department. Once one begins to think systemically, bodily processes become a context for processes of mind and processes of mind for the body. These systems are influencing of and informed by cultural processes. So we see how the systemic view of mutual influence, still a useful concept today, emerges. The beginnings of systemic family therapy emerged from this period and many schools or styles of practice developed up to and including the present day. Our goal is not to provide a detailed account of the history of family therapy (for a comprehensive overview see Dallos & Draper, 2010) but rather to introduce some key historical material and in doing so highlight what characterises systemic thinking and practice more broadly.

An impetus for the move to family- and system-based approaches was the lack of success of individual approaches to psychotherapy, as there were 'many therapists who found that work with an individual did not lead to lasting change once that individual returned to their context/family' (Rivett, 2012, p. 603). This pragmatic search for alternatives was connected with the 'frustration with the failure of the familiar psychodynamic and psychoanalytic approaches ... with difficult-to-manage adolescents and some seriously disturbed psychotic individuals' (Anderson, 1997, p. 15). Working with the family (at this stage of the field this was the system in focus) widened the view of therapists and their perceived sphere of influence. Although much early work was focused on locating and correcting dysfunction the first theorists began with a respectful approach:

> Bateson and others argued that human systems are more likely to change if the therapist respected the integrity of the system (e.g. the way relationship patterns balanced each other) and introduced difference into the system by altering meanings, behaviours or feelings.
>
> (Rivett, 2012, p. 603)

Multiple descriptions, having more than one description of the 'same' event, was a way of introducing something new to the family system. One could not know what this was if one did not spend time getting to know and having a respect for the way the system operated. For therapists, systemic thinking was nothing less than a paradigm shift as the focus moved from what was occurring in the mind of an individual to what was happening between a system of individuals, and this had the implication that 'as family dynamics change, so individual identity and experience can change alongside it' (Dallos & Draper, 2010, p. 31). For a systemic approach, pointing towards one person in a system as 'the problem' was not only unhelpful in supporting useful therapeutic change but also even the attempt at therapy could be ethically problematic once a systems view was developed. This was the problem of scapegoating one family member for the difficulties in the family system, as Dallos and Draper (2010, p. 31) note: 'particularly for children and other disempowered family members, it [a systemic approach] offered a lifeline from the double abuse of being oppressed by the family dynamics and simultaneously being stigmatized for the consequences experienced.' Early systemic family therapy approaches focused on a functional view of problems. Dallos and Draper (2010, pp. 31–32) provide an example of parents quarrelling and their child showing symptoms (e.g. anxiety or acting out). These symptoms then serve the function of distracting the parents from their rows and the family achieves some kind of balance. The family may, in the words of the cliché, develop the idea that they are staying together for the child. In a sense the child has learnt to be ill and this is an important notion for systemic thinking: how are people learning to act in this way or that, feel what they feel, think the way the think, respond and become who they are becoming? The symptoms of the child's illness are required by the family (and may benefit the child also); however, the child is also scapegoated by this and viewed as containing the pathology, thus being the root cause of the 'problem'.

These early approaches also took an 'expert position', tending to see the therapist's role as to look for problems in the family system and attempt to correct them. For example, strategic therapy focused on 'how families could become stuck in repetitive loops of unfulfilling behaviour or in hierarchical structures that were improperly balanced, and what therapists could do to interrupt those patterns and guide families into a healthy rather than unhealthy stability' (Freedman & Combs, 1996, p. 3). This early expert and objective phase is often described as first order, or the first wave of family systemic therapy.

Therapists, influenced by feminist critiques (see McConaghy & Cottone, 1998) highlighting ethical issues with circular causality (for example the morally concerning circular logic that might view perpetrators and victims of domestic violence as locked into mutually reinforcing patterns) as a form of victim blaming, and constructivist scientists such as Humberto Maturana, Francisco Varela and Heinz von Foerster, became less certain that one could have objective knowledge of a system. For constructivists one could have an experience of a system's experience but not an objective account of it. This leads back to early theorists such as Alfred Korzybski, who declared that the map is not the territory. All we have are maps.

As Rivett describes: 'These therapies are called "second order" because they acknowledge that the therapist could never be an expert on the family system. He or she could only describe what their experience was of that system.' (Rivett, 2012, p. 6) This being so, the systemic therapist becomes a member of the therapeutic system and 'couldn't really stand outside the family systems to make "objective" assessments and adjustments' (Freedman & Combs, 1996, p. 5).

This shift brought an altered relationship with aspects of power in the therapeutic system – issues such as child abuse and domestic violence were able to be seen in a context that was not merely within and of the family system, and the therapist was viewed as 'an active, necessarily biased, co-constructor of therapeutic realities' (Campbell, 2003, p.18).

In his consideration of the gifts or 'bounty' of the Milan approach to systemic psychotherapy, Campbell (2003) proffered four key areas that he considered to have evolved from their original contribution: the systemic interview; the use of teams of practitioners to offer a wider range of ideas and reflections; understanding of context; and the use of self in developing a therapeutic relationship. In this paper he gave an excellent, though necessarily brief, account of the evolution of each of these. He went on to develop an analysis of 'newer' ideas from the Milan perspective, which he identified as social constructionism; language and meaning; narrative; integrative models; and work with organisations. Just a few years later, when Hoffman (2006) reflected on her 'three pillars of wisdom' that 'anchor' the work of her systemic psychotherapeutic community she also identified 'reflecting teams' (Andersen, 1987) or, to use Goolishian's preferred term, 'reflecting process', in addition to a 'not-knowing stance' (Anderson & Goolishian, 1988; Anderson, 2001) and 'witnessing process' (Hoffman, 2006).

Cecchin (1987) developed the idea of neutrality, in which a practitioner avoids favouring any particular idea, into curiosity, an exploration of the ideas of both the family and therapist. An extension of this saw the evolution of the concepts of Irreverence (Cecchin et al.,1992) and, later, Prejudice (Cecchin et al.,1994). The latter idea, as a way to consider the biases and ideas that the therapist brings to the therapeutic system, has become embedded in systemic practice. In developing the work on irreverence, Cecchin et al. were endeavouring to respond to the debates they thought were then prevalent in the systemic community regarding models, theories and 'which school of therapy is "more correct"' (1992, p. xiii).

Irreverence works to encourage the therapist to relinquish the restrictions upon what is possible that might be imposed by having a particular approach, school or model, and enables the therapist to consider if there is an alternative way of working with a client or hypothesising about the issues of the family they are considering. It requires us to think about all the possible ways of achieving something and recognising in what direction we are inclined to go so that we are not habitual in our actions. Cecchin et al. (1994) reclaimed the term 'prejudices' to incorporate any fixed view, idea or knowledge that a person holds. This freed up the reader to consider these aspects of their thinking without being caught in a cycle of confusion or doubt. Cecchin et al. (2010) took up 'eccentricity and intolerance' to explore how therapists might avoid the language of pathology and focus instead on the language of eccentricity, witnessing unusual client stories and the sense they might make in the complex contexts in which they exist. This work also highlighted the, often contradictory, contexts of the mental health worker:

> On the one hand, the mental health worker who suffers under the beneficial illusion that their purpose is to help, educate, protect, and cure people, are on the other hand paid by governmental entities of the society who are mainly interested in controlling, segregating and being defended from the social deviant.

> (Cecchin et al., 2010, p. 8)

A third period, also called a 'wave', is noted in the literature and is characterised by terms such as 'postmodernism' and 'social constructionism'. Brown (2010) proposed that the combination of an emphasis on collaboration (Hoffman, 1993), Anderson and Goolishian's (1988) 'not-knowing stance' and postmodern critique (challenging the idea that there is one true reality and exploring how systemic therapy was constructed) catalysed systemic therapy into the next stage of its development. Indeed, Anderson later identified her approach as 'postmodern collaborative' (2001). The further development of Coordinated Management of Meaning, a theory developed initially by Barnett Pearce and Vernon Cronen in the 1970s (Cronen & Lang, 1994; Pearce, 2007; Cronen et al., 2009), and Anderson and Goolishian's (1988) suggestion that human systems are systems in language – the linguistic systems paradigm – were key concepts in this third postmodern phase of systemic therapy. The approaches foreground the notion that social realities are made in communication and when we engage in conversations with clients; when we notice or pass over; how we interpret; the questions we ask, and those we do not, all contribute to the construction of meanings with a client who also influences us with their interpretations and responses. Fredman sums it up thus: 'we construct our realities in conversations and relationships with others and ... these realities are constituted through language and maintained through narratives' (2006, p. 8). This process of knowledge construction takes place across time and cultures in individual conversations and episodes of communication and as reflected in wider cultural change. As we shall see in the following chapter, knowledge concerning learning disability has changed over time, manifested at levels from policy (from institutionalisation to inclusion) to our day-to-day interactions (from service-focused practice to person-centred practice). In this third phase many therapists rejected what they saw as an expert and controlling style of therapy. Psychologist John Shotter worked with and wrote about the work of psychiatrist and systemic therapist Tom Andersen, and noted the change for him in the late 1980s. Tom felt that in his practice at the time he was in effect 'saying, you should stop thinking like you do, and start thinking like us; it was about telling other people how they should live their lives. They could not continue with it' (in Shotter, 2011, p. 637). For Gergen (1999) there was now a focus on meaning as well as interaction and the stories that people live and bring with them to therapy. Therapy becomes a co-construction as therapist and clients create meanings and stories together in their work. There is a focus on relationship, which arguably has always been a part of systemic thinking, and attention to value sensitivity including issues of power and social difference. Contemporary systemic practice draws on this tradition of work, focusing on the space between people, their stories, patterns of interaction, and stories about patterns of interaction. It is no longer oriented by a search for dysfunction and a belief that a therapist's view can be objective, but rather it seeks to collaborate with those who consult with us to co-create desired changes. Writing about systemic therapy in the context of mental health, Professor Peter Stratton noted: 'It does not see its work as being to cure mental illnesses that reside within individuals, but to help people to mobilise the strengths of their relationships so as to make disturbing symptoms unnecessary or less problematic.' (Stratton, 2011, p. 5)

In current systemic literature there appears to be a willingness to move away from the social constructionist theory that had arguably underpinned systemic psychotherapy since the 1980s. Brown suggests that the dialogical approach may be the *fourth order* of family therapy:

> At the core of the dialogical approach is a movement past the focus on words into the realm of 'the between' as revealed in the therapeutic dialogue.
>
> (Brown, 2010)

In this phase, considerations of embodied knowing and communication are coming to the fore (Flaskas et al., 2005). Rober (2005) argued that Anderson's 'not-knowing' stance requires therapists to include reflecting upon their own experience and internal conversation and consider what this has to offer the therapeutic conversation. Anderson (2005) countered that this is indeed what her work with dialogical therapy and processes of the therapist's 'inner dialogical space' (1997) had already achieved.

Bringing the consideration of positions (such as male/female or mother/daughter) into therapeutic process makes it possible to bring power relations and aspects of dominant social discourse into the therapeutic conversation through the narrative of the individual's experience (Winslade, 2005). Campbell and Gronbaek (2006) explored techniques that utilise positioning when they articulated a model that explicitly identified, organised and talked about positions with their clients.

More than 25 years ago Anderson and Goolishian (1992) were using the idea that therapists should position themselves with regard to what they know and what they think they know. They suggested that we should assume a position, or stance, of 'not-knowing' and considered this an ethical position to take that incorporated always holding their 'therapist knowing open to question and change' (p. 350). Positioning is now being used to influence the training of systemic psychotherapists, who are invited to consider how they position themselves epistemologically (Dickerson, 2010). Thus, the development of positioning has influenced how we can see the client, therapist and therapeutic process by listening to our inner voice. For example we ask ourselves: *as a male therapist how I am hearing this client? As a father and son how am I hearing them? What discourses (gender/disability/race?) might be supporting this interpretation? How could I listen differently? If I listened for strengths and abilities how would that change the meanings in the conversation? If I listened out for signs of a diagnosis what would I find and what would I miss? What positions am I being offered when a family tells me they could attend the session with their son if I feel it would be useful?* Positioning is not always intentional; we are positioned by self and others and this occurs in the language we use.

Box 1.3 How are you reading this book?

How are you reading this book?

What is foregrounded in your reading and when? Your gender, status as disabled or non-disabled, your profession or perhaps your class?

Are you creating connections with your experiences and the text? Looking out for gaps and problems with the text? Seeking out the aspects of this text that you might come to value and develop for yourself?

Summary

In summary, Brown (2010) identified 'a conceptual map' of the evolution of the original Milan principles (hypothesising, circularity and neutrality) through the development of systemic approaches. She suggested that there are four stages of systemic focus and practice: Milan (action); post-Milan (stance);

postmodern (orientation) and dialogical (the between). She proposed that each stage benefited from a catalyst, which sped up the reaction into the new phase. Respectively these are: change, power, collaboration and 'the challenge'. Each stage of systemic focus and practice has benefited from the repeated application and reapplication of the concepts and techniques of: questioning (e.g. Tomm, 1987a, 1987b, 1988); curiosity (Cecchin, 1987); not-knowing (Anderson & Goolishian, 1988); and understanding (e.g. Strong & Tomm, 2007).

References

Andersen, T. (1987). The reflecting team: Dialogue and meta-dialogue in clinical work. *Family Process, 26,* 415–428.

Anderson, H. (1997). *Conversation, Language, and Possibilities: A Postmodern Approach to Therapy.* New York: Basic Books.

Anderson, H. (2001). Postmodern collaborative and person-centred therapies: What would Carl Rogers say? *Journal of Family Therapy, 23,* 339–360.

Anderson, H. (2005). Myths about 'not-knowing'. *Family Process, 44*(4), 497–504.

Anderson, H. & Goolishian, H. (1988). Human systems as linguistic systems: Evolving ideas for the implications in theory and practice. *Family Process, 27,* 371–393.

Anderson, H. & Goolishian, H. (1992). The client is the expert: A not-knowing approach to therapy. In S.E. McNamee & K.J. Gergen, *Therapy as Social Construction* (pp. 25–39). London: Sage.

Bateson, N. (2016). *Smaller Arcs of Larger Circles.* Axminster, UK: Triarchy Press.

Brown, J. (2010). The Milan principles of hypothesising, circularity and neutrality in dialogical family therapy: Extinction, evolution, eviction … or emergence? *Australia and New Zealand Journal of Family Therapy, 31*(3), 248–265.

Campbell, D. (2003). The mutiny and the bounty: The place of Milan ideas today. *Australia and New Zealand Journal of Family Therapy, 24*(1), 15–25.

Campbell, D. & Gronbaek, M. (2006). *Taking Positions in the Organisation.* London: Karnac.

Cecchin, G. (1987). Hypothesizing-circularity-neutrality revisited: An invitation to curiosity. *Family Process, 26,* 405–413.

Cecchin, G., Lane, G. & Ray, W. (1992). *Irreverence. A Strategy for Therapists' Survival.* London: Karnac.

Cecchin, G., Lane, G. & Ray, W. (1994). *The Cybernetics of Prejudices in the Practice of Psychotherapy.* London: Karnac.

Cecchin, G., Lane, G. & Ray, W. (2010). Eccentricity and intolerance: A systemic critique. *Human Systems, 21*(1), 7–26.

Charlton, N.G. (2008). *Understanding Gregory Bateson: Mind, Beauty, and the Sacred Earth.* New York: SUNY Press. Retrieved from http://ebookcentral.proquest.com.

Cooperrider, D.L. & Srivastva, S. (1987). Appreciative inquiry in organizational life. *Research in Organizational Change and Development, 1*(1), 129–169.

Cronen, V. & Lang, P. (1994) Language and action: Wittgenstein and Dewey in the practice of therapy and consultation. *Human Systems, 5*(1), 5–43.

Cronen, V., Lang, P. & Lang, S. (2009). Circular questions and coordinated management of meaning theory. *Human Systems, 20*(1), 7–34.

Dallos, R. & Draper, R. (2010). *An Introduction to Family Therapy: Systemic Theory and Practice.* Buckingham: McGraw-Hill Education.

Dickerson, V.C. (2010). Postioning oneself within an epistemology: Refining our thinking about integrative approaches. *Family Process, 49*(3), 349–368.

Flaskas, C., Mason, B. & Perlesz, A. (eds) (2005). *The Space Between: Experience, Context and the Process in the Therapeutic Relationship (Systemic Thinking and Practice).* London: Karnac.

Fredman, G. (2006). Working systemically with intellectual disability: Why not? In S. Baum & H.E. Lynggaard (eds), *Intellectual Disabilities: A Systemic Approach* (pp. 1–20). London: Karnac.

Freedman, J. & Combs, G. (1996). *Narrative Therapy: The Social Construction of Preferred Realities.* London: W.W. Norton & Company.

Gergen, K.J. (1999). *An Invitation to Social Construction.* Thousand Oaks: Sage.

Hedges, F. (2005). *An Introduction to Systemic Therapy with Individuals: A Social Constructionist Approach.* Basingstoke: Palgrave Macmillan.

Hoffman, L. (1993). *Exchanging Voices A Collaborative Approach to Family Therapy.* London: Karnac.

Hoffman, L. (2006). Practising 'withness': A human art. In H. Anderson & P. Jensen (eds), *Innovations in the Reflecting Process 2007* (pp. 3–15). London: Karnac.

Holford, K. (2017). Systemic Haiku. *Murmurations: Journal of Transformative Systemic Practice, 1*(1), 80–83. https://doi.org/10.28963/1.1.8.

Lang, P. & McAdam, E. (2001). Meetings for the first time: Making connections, openings to the best way forward. Family and network consultations. Unpublished manuscript, Kensington Consultation Centre, London.

Lay, L. & Kirk, L. (2014). Person-Centred Strategies for Planning. In H. Atherton & D. Crickmore (eds), *Learning Disabilities – e-book: Towards Inclusion* (pp. 145–159). Retrieved from https://ebookcentral.proquest.com.

McConaghy, J.S. & Cottone, R.R. (1998). The systemic view of violence: An ethical perspective. *Family Process, 37*, 51–63.

Murray, P. (2005). Being in school: Disabled children and the denial of psychological reality. In D. Goodley & R. Lawthom, *Disability and Psychology: Critical Introductions and Reflections* (pp. 34–41). London: Palgrave Macmillan.

Pearce, W.B. (2007). *Making Social Worlds: A Communication Perspective.* Thousand Oaks, CA: Blackwell.

Pearce, W.B. (2011) At Home in the Universe with Miracles and Horizons: Reflections on Personal and Social Evolution. V 3.1, March 23, 2011. http://pearceassociates.com/essays/documents/AtHomeintheUniversewithMiraclesandHorizonsv3-1.pdf (accessed 7 January 2019).

Rivett, M. (2012). Family and systemic therapy. In C. Feltham and I. Horton (eds), *Sage Handbook of Counselling and Psychotherapy*, 3rd edition, 602–607.

Rober, P. (2005). The therapist's self in dialogical family therapy: Some ideas about not-knowing and the therapist's inner conversation. *Family Process*, 44(4), 477–494.

Shotter, J. (2011). Not to forget Tom Andersen's way of being Tom Andersen: The importance of what 'just happens' to us. *Human Systems*, 22(2), 627–652.

Stratton, P. (2011). *The Evidence Base of Family Therapy and Systemic Practice*. United Kingdom: Association for Family Therapy. www.aft.org.uk/SpringboardWebApp/userfiles/aft/file/Research/Evidence-base.pdf (accessed 24 August 2018).

Strong, T. & Tomm, K. (2007). Family therapy as re-coordinating and moving on together. *Journal of Systemic Therapies*, Summer, 26(2), 42–54.

Tomm, K. (1987a). Interventive interviewing: I. Strategizing as a fourth guideline for the therapist. *Family Process*, 26, 3–13.

Tomm, K. (1987b). Interventive interviewing: II. Reflexive questioning as a means to enable self-healing. *Family Process*, 26, 167–83.

Tomm, K. (1988). Interventive interviewing: III. Intending to ask circular, strategic or reflexive questions?. *Family Process*, 27, 1–15.

Winslade, J.M. (2005). Utilising discursive positioning in counselling. *British Journal of Guidance and Counselling*, 33(3), August, 351–364.

2

What is Social Construction and What Does it Offer Learning Disability Scholarship and Practice?

Karl Nunkoosing

Accessible summary

- This chapter explains how different groups of powerful people agree what is knowledge about learning disability. This way of understanding is called *social construction*. Social construction points out that people with learning disability are rarely given a role in making this knowledge. They should be, because this is about their lives.

- There are ways to question the knowledge about learning disability of staff, professionals and people in universities. The chapter explains what these questions are.

- One of the ideas here is that no one is born learning disabled. It is some-thing that professionals say you are. People may be treated badly when others say they are disabled. This is called stigma. Disabled people learn to deal with this stigma.

- We can look for the talents and gifts of disabled people, not just what is 'wrong' with them. Services and staff may keep people with disabilities under watch. Professionals, staff and services can think about their work in new ways so that they can make new relationships with people.

Introduction

You know how to read. What would you say if I suggest that there is more than one way to read a text? My social constructionist bent suggests that I should beware of any text, talk, image, idea or concept that presents itself as the truth. There is no one all-embracing truth; there must always be doubt. Some people, whether policy makers or a powerful organisation that seeks to regulate our knowledge and action, might present their take on whatever topic as fact. You, the reader, have the authority to disagree with the author. This also applies to what you are going to read in this chapter. Think about how some of the knowledge that we take for granted now will become the fallacy of the future. Until recently we quite happily thought of gender in terms of the binary male/female. Of course some people are discomforted by our understanding of sexual orientation in terms of LGBT (lesbian, gay, bisexual and transsexual). Consider why these people take this stance and what argument (and opinions) they might muster to justify their claims. When you do that, you are reading critically. Criticality is at the root of the social constructionist way of understanding.

So, as you read this chapter I ask that you evaluate the ideas I present here. Yes, 'evaluate' means asking what the value is of whatever one is considering. As a social constructionist I acknowledge that there is no single truth, and that there are competing truths, there are multiple truths. I still read/hear about how segregated schooling serves the education of learning disabled children better than inclusive schools.

When you come across my points-ideas-assertions-opinions you are of course at liberty to disagree with me. However, since this book is about systemic approaches I ask you to ask yourself why you find the point-idea-assertion-opinion so disagreeable.

When we say that learning disability is socially constructed, we acknowledge its existence and that how we conceive of it changes over time and across contexts. Currently we have several identities of learning disability, such as 'developmental disability', 'intellectual disability' and 'learning difficulty'. Historically we have used nomenclatures such as 'mentally handicapped' and 'mental deficiency'. These name changes are supposedly reflections of social changes in values and attitude. However, before values and attitudes change, knowledge has to change. To what extent have our values and attitudes changed when we continue to ignore the advice of the self-advocacy movement that we should use the term 'people with learning difficulties'?

There are several points in the short paragraph above that illustrate features of the social constructionist approach identified by Gergen (1985):

1. A critical stance towards knowledge that is taken for granted.

2. Historical and cultural specificity of knowledge.

3. Knowledge and action go together, language itself is a social action.

I shall be attending to these features of the constructionist perspective further in this chapter. Rather than writing about what the social construction of learning disability is, I shall be writing about how my understanding of social constructionism contributes to my take on those we refer to as 'learning disabled people'.

The *critical stance* directs me to point out that people who experience learning difficulties do not appear to have a role in deciding what they are called. That authority is given to the professionals, the academics and the policy makers. On its webpage 'Information about learning disabilities' (www.bild.org. uk/resources/faqs), the British Institute of Learning Disability (BILD) acknowledges that 'people with learning difficulties' is the preferred language of the self-advocacy movement. The unstated reason/s for ignoring this preference is that whilst BILD is a worthy organisation, it represents professionals and academics of learning disability rather than the people who experience learning difficulties. In addition to the 'critical stance', I would also point out how language is a form of social action. The advocacy movement does not exercise the same 'power' as the representatives of learning disability academia and professionals. These language changes indicate how our knowledge of 'learning disability' has changed and the 'critical stance' indicates that this is knowledge that will change in the future. That is why the language that we make available and accessible to ourselves when we discourse 'learning disability' is a choice that we have. In part this is what is meant by language as social action. It will be our critical stance on the taken for granted that is and will be the impetus for new knowing and ways of knowing that are more likely to serve the interests of people who experience learning difficulties, and their supporters.

A critical stance is not about criticising. It is a position that one takes. It starts by asking questions about knowledge/ideas/concepts/policies, such as:

> ➤ What purpose and whose purpose does this theory or policy or practice serve?

> ➤ What does this mean to the man or woman who experiences 'learning disability'?

> ➤ Whose power is being enhanced by this idea/theory/concept/policy/ practice?

> ➤ Whose power is being left undisturbed by this idea/theory/concept/policy/ practice?

> ➤ What do people who experience learning difficulties want from this idea/ theory/concept/policy/practice?

> ➤ Who benefits the most from this idea/theory/concept/policy/practice?

Box 2.1 Questions to encourage 'critical' thinking

What do you know about the lives of the persons that you support who experience learning difficulties?

Who are people who experience learning difficulties and what do they want?

When and how do we explain the theories that inform us about our work to the people who depend on our expertise?

How are you going to explain to the people who experience learning difficulties what a systemic approach means?

How does the culture of your workplace construct issues of race-ethnicity of persons with learning difficulties?

How is a person's sexuality being discoursed in your workplace?

How does this workplace culture construct the abilities of the persons it serves?

A critical stance allows us to judge the extent that our adherence to notions of morality, fairness and justice guide our day-to-day dealings and relationships with men and women who experience learning difficulties who depend on our support.

Social constructionism has the potential to enable us to think differently about theory, practice and policies and their influences regarding our relationships with the persons who experience learning difficulties. Central to this endeavour is to consider/question the objectivity of our knowledge of learning disability. I contend that there is no objective measure of learning disability because it is a product of cultures rather than something that is biological, something that exists inside the person. 'Learning disabled' is an acquired status that is conferred on the labelled person as a result of social and cultural transactions. One does not become learning disabled by oneself. This is a status that is conferred onto a person by a host of psychological, educational and medical professionals. The knowledge-power of these institutions is based on agreed consensus of practices, such as the tests used for the assessment of the intellect and social competence. These tests are based on theories which are agreed upon, that is socially constructed, by academic-practitioners, and are employed to make validity and reliability claims to legitimise their use. The tests often assume that 'learning disability' resides inside the person.

When we say that knowledge of learning disability is socially constructed, we infer that what we know, and take for granted, is the result of our everyday engagements with others who make claims to knowing about learning disability. We give authority to our textbooks and their authors. As students we, often uncritically, construct our own texts with fragments of texts from these worthies in order to get good marks for our essays. We call upon their authority when we make a case for either our research or our practice. We thus become part of the social network that gives social construction its name. Social construction is thus the act of talking and writing, of contributing to narratives of our work and our relationships with men and women, boys and girls who have, for now, been given the status of 'learning disabled' and 'intellectually disabled' in some cultures with equally credible knowledge claims, and 'mentally handicapped' at some past time in our history. There are men and women living today who in their lifetime have been referred to as subnormal, handicapped, and disabled. Imagine what that does to one's identity!

The history of people who experience learning difficulties is also our history. Much of this history has not been written or told by people who experience learning difficulties. This is changing; there is now a corpus of data about the experiences of self-advocates, and a growing literature about the, often combative, experiences of parents of sons and daughters who experience learning difficulties. Self-advocates provide another community that can potentially add to the social construction of learning disability. When we listen to these voices we will hear much of what is wrong with services and their employees: what is wrong with what we do; with how we do what we do; and with our relationships with the people we are meant to serve.

Box 2.2 Constructing Knowledge. Consider...

Consider how we are going to stop marginalising the knowledge of self-advocates and parent-advocates in the construction of learning disability knowledge.

Earlier I raised the issue about how one becomes or gets given the spoilt identity (Goffman, 1963) 'learning disabled'. In their study of people who have been given the label/spoilt identity/diagnosis of 'learning disability', Finlay and Lyons (2000) found that the participants who experience learning difficulties neither identify themselves nor refer to themselves by this label. They do so because they are aware of the stigma (Goffman, 1990) associated with this label, 'learning disability'. In our supportive and educational work with persons who experience learning difficulties we need to attend to enabling them to understand the influence of stigma of learning disability on their lives. We may know about stigma, we may talk/discuss, do seminars and write essays about it. However, in what ways do we attend to this theory in our day-to-day dealings with people who risk stigmatisation? If we don't, why might that be? Is it possible that we experience what Goffman (1963) calls 'courtesy stigma' and describes as 'the tendency for stigma to spread from the stigmatised individual to his close connections' (p. 30)?

That is stigma experienced by persons who associate with people who are stigmatised.

However, our obsession with the pathological is such that when we research or read about the life experiences of men and women who experience learning difficulties, we zoom in on the experience of isolation, rejection and abuse. We should also attend to their narratives of resilience and survival despite the often lifelong adversities they encounter as they negotiate their identities (Horn & Moss, 2015).

So our denial of the presence and influence of the stigmatised and discrediting status of the person who experiences learning difficulties may be a way of dealing with our courtesy stigma. In a series of discourse analytical research studies my colleague Treena Jingree (Jingree et al., 2006; Jingree & Finlay, 2008, 2013) has demonstrated how service workers muster a range of discursive strategies to discount the narratives of men and women in their care who experience learning disabilities. Participants distinguished between choice in theory and in practice, with practice constructed as impractical. In constructing persons with learning disability making choices as impracticable, participants saw the problems arising from the inability of the disabled person. This is a disabling discourse. The critical constructionist take here is that the inability resides in the workers' lack of competencies to enable people who experience learning difficulties to exercise choice, not in the inability of the learning disabled person to exercise choice. This is in effect a good example of the social model of disability idea that people are not disabled by their impairment; they are disabled by society and, in Jingree's work, by the people who are meant to support them.

So how is it that people whom one might expect to defend the 'rights' of people who experience learning difficulties harbour beliefs, that they might say are realistic, that are so devoid of hope that they are discriminatory? Deal (2007) proposed the concept of 'aversive disablism' to illustrate the point that people who have learnt that overt disablist attitudes, prejudices and discrimination towards disabled people are wrong do not recognise themselves as prejudiced and yet may harbour prejudicial beliefs and consequently engage in disablist practices.

I suggest that some learning disabled people's reactions to stigma are labelled as challenging behaviours. An aspect of the stigma of learning disability is that service workers tend to postulate the cause of people's action as being located in their heads rather than in the relational system they live in. Whilst not directly referring to stigma, Haydon-Laurelut and Nunkoosing (2010) provide an example of how attention to the relational can evoke a richer story by reimagining what gets labelled as challenging behaviour as having its cause in a troubled relationship between a man who experiences learning difficulties and the service workers who support him. Such reimagining is going to be hard where the predominant culture of a service is influenced by 'deficit thinking' (Valencia, 1997) where the problems that 'learning disabled' persons encounter are caused by their impairments. In a study of five youngsters with learning disabilities in inclusive classrooms, Smith (2000) observed how some teachers are so steeped in the paradigm of the incompetence of the labelled child that they either fail to notice the achievements of some children or they discount such achievement when it occurs. How is it that the same child is learning disabled in some classes, for some lessons, and not so in other classes? 'Disability is constructed by the meaning people place on it' (Smith, 2000, p. 910).

People who are labelled as 'learning disabled' are aware of the stigma that is attached to this spoilt status. In a study with seven men and one woman aged between 25 and 63 who were newly diagnosed as having a learning disability, Kenyon et al. (2014) found that the participants were fully aware of how they are stigmatised. The participants had also developed strategies to deal with these experiences. You could ask why these persons were described as 'newly diagnosed'. Kenyon et al. (2014) reported that they were mostly diagnosed whilst at school but had not been diagnosed since they were 18. The interesting thing is that they had lived their adult lives without the label/diagnosis, which begs the question of why they were brought to the attention of agencies that led to them being diagnosed. If we assume that people who experience learning difficulties do not know that the label 'learning disabled' is stigmatising we are simply perpetuating the myth that these people have 'no sense'. This is a version of ableism (Campbell, 2009). If you think that this is somehow far-fetched, ask yourself why our support for persons who experience learning difficulties rarely include how to deal with stigma.

In an interesting study about students with learning disabilities' discourses of challenging behaviour, Lee and Connolly (2016) established that 'challenging behaviours' are discoursed as rational responses to institutional environments. The participant-students with learning disabilities are also aware that the sense that they make of their challenging behaviours is different and in opposition to the theories and explanations of practitioners.

How does one become learning disabled?

Here the work of the influential French philosopher Michel Foucault (1978, 1979) is useful. There are several ways of looking, referred to as 'gazes', that can be brought into action to define a person as abnormal, ill in the head, delinquent or criminal. All these serve as preludes to define the person as suitable to be brought into the punitive and disciplinary gaze of power. The technical gazes of psychology and medicine are associated with the idea of learning disability as pathology. The discourse of power-knowledge of medicine and psychology produces and legitimises knowledge of disability and learning disability. Meanings get attached to these knowledge claims which then produce the actions that people with learning disability become subjected to. The conferred discredited status of being learning disabled justifies the surveillance of people who experience learning difficulties.

Services are in the business of the surveillance of citizens who have been brought to the notice of the service by various social structures in education, health, social care and the justice system. There are, in effect, many more people who experience learning difficulties but have not been brought to the gaze of the learning disability professionals. That is, they are not in need of surveillance. Thus service providers are entrepreneurs who design and implement services that are acceptable to their funders. The services have to continue to maintain the need for surveillance by either portraying the learning disabled person as a victim or as a threat to society. Learning disability professionals and their employers are entrepreneurs who also seek to expand the scope of their activities to colonise more and more aspects of the learning disabled person's life. One of the problems here was pointed out a long time ago by Erving Goffman (1990): service systems invent explanations that make the person in need of support and subject to surveillance.

Such explanations, derived from professional knowledge-power and filtered down to service direct care workers, are products of the medical model of individual impairments of the person's intellect. This runs counter to the social model (Oliver, 1983, 1990) notion that disability, as distinct from impairment, has its origin in the historically discriminatory processes of our society. The problem of the disablement of men and women who experience learning difficulties is often located in the services, the professional and lay employees of the learning disability industry. The disablement of learning difficulties has its origin in our attitude, our lack of hopefulness about the outcome of our support (Nunkoosing & Haydon-Laurelut, 2013), our lack of skill, our unwillingness to make common cause with disabled people, our inability to stop othering the person with learning disability, our inability to see the toxicity of our thinking and actions and our ready willingness to find excuses to justify our power-knowledge. What appears to be personal knowledge that each of us acquire has been tested and examined before one has been allowed to join this or that profession or academic tribe, be it nursing or medicine or social work or education or psychology or sociology or social policy or service management.

Knowledge that does not serve our purposes can also be suppressed. I am amazed how learning disability professionals, policy makers, university teachers, managers, and trainers have suppressed knowledge of the principles of social role valorisation (SRV) (Wolfensberger, 2000). Although not without critique (Elks, 1994; Bleasdale, 1996), SRV was influential in the major service developments during the 1980s and 1990s. Interestingly, it was SRV that raised the issue of values in the ideology of services and yet the twenty-first century saw the White Paper 'Valuing People' (Department of Health, 2001) and at the same time the abandonment of any reference to the work of either Wolfensberger or the earlier idea of normalisation (Nirje, 1969). SRV brought to the surface the unconsciousness that controls our relationship with people labelled as 'learning disabled'. It challenged our taken-for-granted views of the congregation and segregation of learning disabled people as something benign, rather than their punitive surveillance. The suppression of SRV is, in effect, a good example of how the knowledge and values of one generation do not get transferred or get suppressed; in the language of social constructionism this is referred to as the 'cultural and historical specificity' of knowledge (Burr, 2003, p. 3). The values that guided our thinking during the 1980s/1990s did not serve the project of the privatisation of caring. SRV was too critical, too ideological, and too challenging of the values that maintained the devalued status of learning disabled people and their need to be under surveillance.

The challenge is that people who are made other, such as disabled people, refugees, rough sleepers, and those with unconventional lifestyles, are devalued. That is, they are not accorded the same worth. The suppression of SRV has not led to us valuing learning disabled people. We have simply stopped listening to the voices that ask why learning disabled people are subject to hate crimes (Richardson et al., 2016; McCarthy, 2017); why the abuse of people with learning disabilities has not stopped (Flynn, 2012); why they do not get access to appropriate health care and die from preventable problems when they are ill (Mencap, 2007; Glover et al., 2017).

Although the uncomfortable discourse of 'social role valorisation' has been successfully eradicated, much of what are considered good or best practices in learning disability services have their origins in SRV (Caruso & Osburn, 2011). 'Valuing People' (2001) identified the following as the appropriate outcomes of good services: rights, independence, choice and inclusion. These are in fact originally derived from SRV by John O'Brien and Connie Lyle O'Brien's 'Five Accomplishments', only the original formulation included the encouragement of valued social roles (1998). We have to ask ourselves why the encouragement of valued social roles is so difficult and unpromising that it does not figure in government policy. Consider, also, the taken-for-granted knowledge that we work with people who experience learning difficulties to promote their independence. In our culture of individualism we intellectually celebrate 'independence' and yet live our lives in networks of relationships; of course some relationships can be toxic and some are empowering (see Nunkoosing & Haydon-Laurelut, 2013). What does 'independence' mean for each person who bares the sometimes invisible, but still discrediting, stigma of 'learning disabled'? What does independence mean when our lives are interconnected? My critical social constructionist stance suggests that the taken-for-granted notion of independence is deceitful because services have a vested interest in holding on to the dependence of learning disabled men and women on the services they provide. What does a person's independence mean if it does not attend to inequality? When we speak of inequality we pay attention to dominative power, which is 'power over' (Pratto, 2016). When the man or woman who experiences learning difficulties resists such domination we see this resistance as challenging behaviour.

Staying with the constructionist stance that language is a form of social action I am drawn to the following familiar discourse: '*He is attention seeking; he is having an outburst; he is having a tantrum; he is having a meltdown; he is kicking off; he is off his head; he has thrown a wobbly.*' Yes, these are common in the language of services when we talk about a learning disabled person's challenging acts. I guess that we can all add to this list. What is behind such discourse? To define these as anger and strong emotion is to acknowledge our shared humanness. It seems to me natural to want attention when one lives in an unnatural environment where one is deprived of human attention. Note also how this language often implies the cause of these acts as being located in the head of the learning disabled actor, that he or she has no control. This is the language of service talk and of stigma.

From the Foucauldian viewpoint, no amount of inclusion is going to stop the stigma and its associated devaluation of the man and woman who is seen as other. People are disciplined to act according to the social identity prescribed for them. This affects both the learning disabled person and the other people he or she is in contact with, including service professionals and other employees. It is the discredited status 'learning disabled' that allows and justifies the actions that people with learning disabilities are subjected to, such as their surveillance. It would seem that we are all trapped by the Foucauldian web of power. However, whilst there is always the option of resistance, service employers would not tolerate such resistance by its employees, so we continue to choose not to make common cause with people who experience learning difficulties. The prelude to such a stance of resistance is our engagement in reflection about our role and actions with and on behalf of people with learning disabilities.

The tension is between how the presence of a learning difficulty makes the man or woman in need of assistance and how this assistance can be provided without surveillance, and with the prospect of enabling him or her to live a good life in a good society. The social model of disability (Oliver, 1983, 1990) suggests that the problems of 'learning disabilities' are not in the individual intellectual impairment but in our attitudes, our lack of technology, our unwillingness to stop othering the person who experiences learning difficulties, and our inability to see the toxicity of our thinking and actions.

What will have to change? With Foucault we understand how professional knowledge-power of learning disability is used for and on behalf of government as a coercive influence to maintain the surveillance of people who get labelled as learning disabled. We do this to achieve social order but we neutralise our collusion by framing our work as helping or as justifying the surveillance of people with learning disabilities. Our employers make the learning disabled person who has come into the notice of services always visible; that is one meaning of surveillance. We should note that much of what gets written about people with learning disabilities is in effect about the minority of people with a learning disability who come to the attention of services.

References

Bleasdale, M. (1996). Evaluating 'values' – A critique of value theory on social role valorisation. *Australian Disability Review*, 1, 3–22.

Burr, V. (2003). *Social Constructionism*, 2nd edition. London: Routledge.

Campbell, F.K. (2009). *Contours of Ableism: The Production of Disability and Ableness*. Basingstoke: Palgrave Macmillan.

Caruso, G.A. & Osburn, J.A. (2011). The origins of 'best practices' in the principle of normalization and social role valorization. *Journal of Policy and Practice in Intellectual Disabilities*, 8, 191–196.

Deal, M. (2007). Aversive disablism: Subtle prejudices towards disabled people. *Disability and Society*, 21, 93–107.

Department of Health. (2001). *Valuing People: A New Strategy for Learning Disability for the 21st Century*. London: Department of Health.

Elks, M. (1994). Valuing the person or valuing the role? Critiques of social role valorization theory. *Mental Retardation*, 32, 265–271.

Finlay, W.M.L. & Lyons, E. (2000). Social categorisation, social comparison and stigma: Presentation of self in people with learning difficulties. *British Journal of Social Psychology*, 39, 129–146.

Flynn, M. (2012). *Winterbourne View Hospital: A Serious Case Review*. Yate: The South Gloucestershire Safeguarding Adults Board, South Gloucestershire Council.

Foucault, M. (1978). *The History of Sexuality Vol 1. An Introduction*. London: Allen Kane.

Foucault, M. (1979). *Discipline and Punish: The Birth of the Prison*. Harmondsworth: Penguin.

Gergen, K.J. (1985). The constructionist movement in modern psychology. *American Psychologist*, 40, 266–275.

Glover, G., Williams, R., Heslop, P., Oyinlola, J. & Grey, J. (2017). Mortality in people with intellectual disabilities in England. *Journal of Intellectual Disability Research*, Jan 61(1), 62–74.

Goffman, E. (1963). *Stigma. Notes on the Management of Spoiled Identity*. New York: Simon and Schuster.

Goffman, E. (1990). *Stigma: Notes on the Management of Spoiled Identity*. Harmondsworth: Penguin.

Haydon-Laurelut, M. & Nunkoosing, K. (2010). 'I want to be listened to': Systemic psychotherapy with a man with intellectual disability and his paid supporters. *Journal of Family Therapy*, 32, 73–86.

Horn, J.H. & Moss, D. (2015). A search for meaning: Telling your life with learning disabilities. *British Journal of Learning Disabilities*, 43, 178–185.

Jingree, T., Finlay, W.M. & Antaki, C. (2006). Empowering words, disempowering actions. *Journal of Learning Disability Research*, 50, 212–226.

Jingree, T. & Finlay, W.M.L. (2008). 'You can't do it…it's theory rather than practice': Staff use of the practice/principle rhetorical device in talk on empowering people with learning disabilities. *Disability and Society*, 19, 705–726.

Jingree, T. & Finlay, W.M.L. (2013). Expressions of dissatisfaction and complaint by people with learning disabilities: A discourse analytical study. *British Journal of Social Psychology*, 52, 255–272.

Kenyon, E., Beail, N. & Jackson, T. (2014) Learning disabilities: Experience of diagnosis. *British Journal of Learning Disabilities*, 42(4), 257–263.

Lee, L. & Connolly, N. (2016). Challenging behavior as a rational response to institutional norms: Analyzing students' discourse on behaviors deemed challenging. *Journal of Constructivist Psychology*, 29, 417–431.

McCarthy, M. (2017). 'What kind of abuse is him spitting in my food?': Reflections on similarities between disability hate crime, so called 'mate' crime and domestic violence against women with learning disabilities. *Disability & Society*, 32(4), 595–600.

Mencap. (2007). *Death by Indifference*. London: Mencap.

Nirje, B. (1969). The normalization principle and its human management implications. In R.B. Kugel & W. Wolfensberger (eds), *Changing Patterns in Residential Services for the Mentally Retarded* (pp. 179–195). Washington, DC: President's Committee on Mental Retardation.

Nunkoosing, K. & Haydon-Laurelut, M. (2013). *The Relational Basis of Empowerment*. Sheffield: Centre for Welfare Reform.

O'Brien, J. & O'Brien, L. (1998). *Implementing Person-Centered Planning*. Toronto: Inclusion Press.

Oliver, M. (1983). *Social Work with Disabled People*. Basingstoke: Macmillan.

Oliver, M. (1990). *The Politics of Disablement*. Basingstoke: Macmillan.

Pratto, F. (2016). On power and empowerment. *British Journal of Psychology*, 55, 1–20.

Richardson, L., Beadle-Brown, J., Bradshaw, J., Guest, C., Malovic, A. & Himmerich, J. (2016). I felt that I deserved it' – Experiences and implications of disability hate crime. *Tizard Learning Disability Review*, 21, 80–88.

Smith, R.M. (2000). Mystery or typical teens? The social construction of academic engagement and disability. *Disability and Society*, 15, 909–922.

Valencia, R.R. (1997). *The Evolution of Deficit Thinking: Educational Thought and Practice*. London: Routledge.

Wolfensberger, W. (2000). A brief overview of social role valorization. *Mental Retardation*, 38, 105–123.

3

Understanding Disabling Barriers Faced by People with Learning Difficulties: The Social Model and Beyond

Donna Reeve

Accessible summary

- Many people with learning difficulties do not see themselves as disabled. This might be because often people think of disability as not being able to walk, or as 'a bad thing'.

- Often, when writers try to make sense of what disability is, they do not talk about how disabled people feel about themselves, or their feelings in general.

- Some barriers can stop people being able to do things. This is called *structural disablism*.

- Some barriers affect how people feel about themselves and who they can be as people. This is called *psycho-emotional disablism*.

- A definition of disablism which includes barriers which affect what people can physically do (structural disablism) and how they feel about themselves (psycho-emotional disablism), therefore, might be more useful when thinking about the lives of people with learning difficulties.

- Examples of structural disablism include not being able to get into a building because there are steps instead of a lift or ramp, and when people do not take the time to explain things clearly or provide information that is easy to understand.

- Examples of psycho-emotional disablism include being made fun of by strangers, bullying and disability hate crime. It is also happens when people take to heart and believe negative messages about the value of the lives of people with learning difficulties that are held by other people in society.

▶

> ◀
> - Many examples of psycho-emotional disablism stem from the experience of discrimination and result from societal prejudices about people with learning difficulties.
>
> - Understanding the impact of psycho-emotional disablism on self-esteem and emotional well-being is important for professionals working with the mental health of people with learning difficulties.

This chapter will start by describing three different approaches to disability – individual model, social model and normalisation. The rest of the chapter will then discuss the implications of the social model of disability and how this view of disability as a socially constructed barrier has relevance for understanding the lives of people with learning difficulties. It will be suggested that recent clarifications of this definition of disability increase the relevance of the social model of disability for this group of disabled people, who often do not see themselves as disabled. In particular the concept of *psycho-emotional disablism* will be introduced which can impact on emotional well-being and self-esteem and so is of particular relevance for health professionals working therapeutically with people with learning difficulties.

As this chapter is written from a disability studies perspective, I will be reflecting how members of the British self-advocacy movement *People First* choose to self-define. Hence I will be using the term 'learning difficulty' rather than 'learning disability' or 'intellectual disability' throughout.

A Disability Equality Training session … many years ago

Twenty years ago I ran a Disability Equality Training (DET) session with a fellow trainer who was a wheelchair user. We had been invited into a day centre to run this session with a small group of people with learning difficulties and what struck me was how they saw themselves, or not, as disabled people. They were very clear that they were not disabled, unlike the two trainers who had physical impairments impacting on mobility. It was the fact that we had difficulties walking, or *doing*, which marked us as disabled in their eyes. However, they did acknowledge that they had difficulties dealing with strangers who would make fun of them in shops. These experiences upset them a lot and left them feeling devalued and dehumanised. Between us we agreed that these were also disabling barriers which impacted on their emotional well-being, namely barriers to *being*.

Models of disability

Over the last 40 years various different models and approaches to disability have been discussed endlessly within academia, influenced by prevailing trends in epistemology and ontology (for more information see Shakespeare, 2014; Thomas, 2007). I will now briefly outline three models of disability and consider the ramifications these have when attempting to understand the lived experience of someone with learning difficulties.

The individual (or medical) model of disability adopts a deficit approach and places the cause of disability on the individual who cannot function 'normally' because of their impairments, namely physical, psychological, or cognitive difference. Therefore the solution to the 'problem' of disability is to change the individual, and the expert in this case is a professional of some kind. Within this framework, someone with a learning difficulty would be seen as being incapable of being a parent *because* they have a learning difficulty and the 'solution' might be sterilisation to prevent pregnancy. Oliver (1990) argues that this individual model of disability is underpinned by 'personal tragedy theory' where disability is viewed as a terrible chance event which happens to rare unfortunate individuals. In this model, disability is associated with dependency and abnormality. Hence the experience of impairment is inherently negative and disabled people are a group to be feared or avoided because they represent an uncomfortable reminder of mortality. The termination of foetuses in the womb shown to have conditions such as spina bifida or Down's Syndrome could be considered as the extreme consequences of these negative views of impairment – the ultimate denial of the right to life. In this model, disability is associated with dependency and abnormality. Finally, it is a view of disability which has strong cultural roots and can influence the attitudes and beliefs of both disabled and non-disabled people, and it still exists in society today.

No doubt influenced by the fight of civil rights groups in the 1960s, during the 1970s and 1980s disabled people started to self-organise into a political movement, challenging the ways in which disability and disabled people were viewed and treated in society. Crucial to the growth of this disabled people's movement was the articulation of a *social* model of disability, in which it was the ways that society was organised that maintained the exclusion of disabled people, rather than their impairments.

Therefore this exclusion was the consequence of inaccessible buildings and transport, discriminatory employment practices and segregated education, to name but a few examples – all due to a failure to consider the access needs of people with impairments, resulting in profound exclusion in all aspects of social life.

The breaking of the causal link between disability and impairment is a crucial difference between the social and individual models of disability and allowed disabled people to fight for social change, disability rights and equality. Consequently, disabled people achieved inclusion through changes to social structures, institutions and the built environment, not through modifying or blaming the individual with the impairment. The social model also fostered the development of a positive disability culture and disability identity through disability pride. Disabled people, rather than professionals, were now seen as the experts on their lives.

As this chapter is about the lives of people with learning difficulties, I need to briefly mention a model of disability which emerged around the same time as the social model. When the British government decided to close the long-term institutions for people with learning difficulties in the 1970s, normalisation, or what became later known as social role valorisation (SRV), was the model adopted to generate a new way of providing services for people with learning difficulties in the community. One of the key aims of this model required people with learning difficulties to adopt 'culturally valued roles' through associating with individuals with 'high social value'. Hence heterosexual relationships were valued over same-sex relationships; relationships with non-disabled people were valued over relationships with other people with learning difficulties. In addition this model maintained the power imbalance between professionals and people with learning difficulties. The outcome of normalisation is that people with learning difficulties are made to conform to what society deems of value, rather than being valued as unique human beings in their own right (Chappell, 1997).

The social model of disability and people with learning difficulties

Whilst the social model of disability has undoubtedly played a significant role in improving the lives of many disabled people since the 1970s, there have been concerns that certain kinds of 'body' are privileged over others. For example huge improvements have been made to improve access to buildings for people with mobility impairments and wheelchair users via the replacement of steps with ramps and lifts. However, less consistent advances have been made in meeting the access needs of people with learning difficulties such as providing information in accessible formats such as Easy Read. Failure to make reasonable adjustments to allow people with learning difficulties to access the same services as other people can have fatal consequences – it has been shown that people with learning difficulties are at risk of premature death because healthcare services do not make reasonable adjustments to ensure that people with learning difficulties receive the same standard of healthcare as the rest of the general population (Tuffrey-Wijne & Hollins, 2014).

One of the criticisms levelled at the social model of disability is that much of the writing about this radical approach to disability has continued to marginalise the voices of those with learning difficulties. So when many disability studies writers consider 'disabled people', it usually means 'people with physical and sensory impairments', with 'learning difficulty' being 'tagged on only as an afterthought within much of the literature generated by the social model' (Chappell et al., 2001, p. 46). Similarly, people with learning difficulties have felt largely excluded from the wider disabled people's movement because of a tendency by those disabled people without learning difficulties to frame the difficulties associated with learning difficulties as being inherent to the impairment (medical model) rather than as socially constructed (social model) (Simone Aspis in Campbell & Oliver, 1996, p. 97). Consequently, the disabled people's movement does not always recognise, or meet the *access needs*, of people with learning difficulties, and the consequence is marginalisation of the voices of this particular group of disabled people from the movement as a whole. In many respects, this is simply another manifestation of the 'hierarchy of impairment' which circulates in society, whereby people with learning difficulties have lower status than those whose impairment affects the body (Deal, 2003), a hierarchy which is internalised by both disabled and non-disabled people.

One important aspect of the disabled people's movement is that of peer support – disabled people supporting each other. People with learning difficulties have been self-advocating for decades – the founding People First organisation, controlled by and for people with learning difficulties, was set up in the UK in 1984 and there are now hundreds of self-advocacy groups throughout the UK. However, there are some important differences between self-advocacy groups and the disabled people's movement. The disabled people's movement emphasises a proud disabled identity, disability culture and the challenging of disabling social, physical and economic barriers to inclusion in society, whereas much of the focus of the self-advocacy movement has been in improving the services received by people with learning difficulties, possibly because of the history of normalisation/SRV mentioned earlier, which was service-based (Chappell et al., 2001). Nonetheless, People First/self-advocacy groups clearly work within a broadly defined social model understanding of disability and support people with learning difficulties to stand up for their rights and to have choice and control in how their lives are run – namely, challenging exclusion from society.

Additionally, how people with learning difficulties self-identify has been at variance with the general direction of the disabled people's movement, where the term 'disabled person' is preferred to 'person with a disability'. This choice reflects the social model of disability, that disabling barriers are caused by society rather than being a property of the individual. By comparison, in 1985 the self-advocacy movement of people with intellectual impairments chose to self-identify as 'people with learning difficulties' (although it should be acknowledged that some groups of people may reject this particular label and choose to self-identify in other ways, for example as 'people from the learning disability community'). The desire to claim this 'person first' identity – 'person with a learning difficulty' rather than 'disabled person' – was a direct challenge to the dehumanising prejudices circulating in society about people with intellectual impairments (a situation which still exists today, unfortunately). It may also have been influenced by the normalisation agenda of the time where the term 'disabled person' would have had negative connotations to people with learning difficulties because of its association with a stigmatised social identity. Here, Joyce clearly distances herself from a disabled identity:

> 'Learning disabilities' – I don't like that, disability makes you believe that we are in wheel chairs and we can't do anything for ourselves, when we can. We've got jobs now, we've got paid jobs.

> (Joyce Kershaw, self-advocate, quoted in Goodley, 2000, pp. 229–230)

However, even if a person with learning difficulties does not see themselves as disabled, others in society still do, and do not hesitate to treat them differently as a consequence.

A social relational definition of disablism: The naming of psycho-emotional disablism

Thomas (2007) has built on the roots of the social model of disability to produce what she terms an *extended social relational definition of disablism*:

> Disablism is a form of social oppression involving the social imposition of restrictions of activity on people with impairments and the socially engendered undermining of their psycho-emotional well-being.

> (Thomas, 2007, p. 73)

Using the term 'disablism' rather than 'disability' is an attempt to frame the oppression faced by people with impairments as in the same area as other forms of social oppression such as sexism, ageism and racism. Here disablism is composed of two forms – structural disablism and psycho-emotional disablism. *Structural disablism* refers to those socially constructed barriers which affect what people can *do*, such as failing to make a building wheelchair accessible or not providing information in accessible formats for people with learning difficulties. These are the barriers that people usually consider when they think of the social model which operates at the material/public level. Whereas *psycho-emotional disablism* refers to socially constructed barriers which affect who people can *be*, impacting on psycho-emotional well-being and sense of self, which operates at a more personal/private level than structural disablism. In other words:

> The oppression that disabled people experience operates on the 'inside' as well as on the 'outside': it is about being made to feel of lesser value, worthless, unattractive, or disgusting as well it is about 'outside' matters such as being turned down for a job because one is 'disabled', not being able to get one's wheelchair into a shop or onto a bus because of steps, or not being offered the chance of a mainstream education because one has 'special needs'.

> (Thomas, 2004, pp. 38–39)

Here Thomas is describing examples of 'inside' forms of oppression (psycho-emotional disablism) compared to 'outside' forms of oppression (structural disablism).

Although the traditional social model of disability does not deny the reality of these psycho-emotional forms of disablism, nonetheless they have been typically overshadowed by the more 'obvious' material barriers. In part, this is because structural barriers are easier to identify, challenge and change compared to removing societal prejudices about disability which underpin psycho-emotional disablism. Psycho-emotional disablism is not inevitable, and varies over time and place and at different stages in someone's life. For example, being tired and in pain can make it harder to deal with someone making fun of you on the bus on that particular day. In addition, disabled people can and do resist this form of disablism, as I will show later. Whilst the impact of psycho-emotional disablism can vary, a structural barrier such as a flight of steps will always disable a wheelchair user – as the disabled comedian Stella Young quips, 'No amount of smiling at a flight of stairs has ever made it turn into a ramp' (Young, 2014).

There are two forms of psycho-emotional disablism (Reeve, 2008, 2014b). *Indirect* psycho-emotional disablism refers to the emotional consequences of dealing with inaccessible physical environments or reasonable adjustments which are 'unreasonable' to use. For example, the embarrassment of having to ask for the key to the accessible toilet at a crowded bar could lead to indirect psycho-emotional disablism. Another example might be the frustration or anger felt by someone with learning difficulties when dealing with a health professional who fails to explain the details of their medical treatment in terms that they understand and feel comfortable with.

The more common *direct* psycho-emotional disablism arises from the relationships that a disabled person has with other people, and refers to 'acts of invalidation' through words, looks and actions which can leave that disabled person feeling ashamed, worthless, vulnerable and inferior. These include being stared at or avoided by strangers as well as being made fun of or taunted by people for being different. Another example happens when someone speaks to the person supporting the disabled person, rather than addressing the disabled person themselves – the 'Does he take sugar?' treatment, which is highly objectifying.

Whilst it is relationships with family, friends, professionals and strangers who can (often inadvertently) disable the person through their words and actions, the phenomenon of *internalised oppression* is another source of direct psycho-emotional disablism. Internalised oppression arises from the relationship a disabled person has with themselves; it can be experienced by any minority group in society and happens when members of that group internalise the prejudices held about them by the majority group in society. In the case of disability, these prejudices are informed by 'ableism', which constructs certain bodies and minds as impaired and hence as lesser, different, undesirable, positioned as 'Other' relative to the unquestioned normative and normate individual (Campbell, 2009). Therefore it could be argued that the term 'internalised oppression' should strictly be referred to as 'internalised ableism' (Campbell, 2009), but this term has yet to gain traction in disability studies.

Elsewhere I have argued that it is important for counsellors and therapists to be aware of the impact of disabling barriers on the emotional well-being of disabled people (Reeve, 2002, 2014a). Akin to emotional abuse, psycho-emotional disablism has a cumulative impact on emotional well-being (Reeve, 2008) – past experiences of name calling and mockery can exacerbate the impact of present-day psycho-emotional disablism. I also suspect that past experiences of trauma and abuse also increase the potential damage done by psycho-emotional disablism because of the overlap in the ways in which shame, existential anxiety and self-esteem are affected by these assaults on the psyche.

Structural disablism in the lives of people with learning difficulties

Many of the structural barriers faced by people with learning difficulties are common to other groups of disabled people: physical barriers which prevent access to buildings and information; attitudinal barriers which lead to social isolation and avoidance by non-disabled people; economic barriers leading to the highest rates of poverty in society for disabled people (Heslop & Gordon, 2014).

People with learning difficulties who also have physical impairments will face the same difficulties in accessing the built environment as other physically disabled people. However, the presence of learning difficulties may impact on how effective the 'solutions' are for this particular group of disabled people. For example, the ability to drive can provide independence for a wheelchair user but this option is not usually available for someone with a learning difficulty. People with learning difficulties experience disproportionate rates of sensory loss but these sensory impairments are often overlooked by a carer, which means that suitable compensatory aids are not supplied to that person (Emerson & Baines, 2011).

Shakespeare (2014) discusses the impossibility of creating a world which is completely free of structural disablism. For example, in the case of employment, even if all barriers and discrimination were removed, some groups of disabled people such as those with learning difficulties would still find it relatively difficult to find paid employment because of the demand for literacy and numeracy skills in a knowledge economy. Instead it is suggested that this group of disabled people should be offered alternatives to employment which nonetheless provide a 'sense of value, purpose and fulfilment to their lives' (Shakespeare, 2014, p. 42).

Whilst structural disablism can be an important aspect for many people with learning difficulties, it is the impact of psycho-emotional disablism which I now want to consider for the rest of this chapter.

Psycho-emotional disablism in the lives of people with learning difficulties

As I described at the start of this chapter, many people with learning difficulties do not identify as disabled per se. In part this is because of the chosen 'person with a learning difficulty' identity, but also because the signifier for disability, the logo of a wheelchair, reinforces the notion that disabled people have difficulties *doing* something physical such as walking. However, as was clear from discussions with the participants in my DET session, whilst this group of people with learning difficulties could manage to negotiate the built environment – they didn't experience *structural disablism* – nonetheless they were upset by the ways that strangers in shops would humiliate them – they did experience *psycho-emotional disablism*.

Hence using a definition of disablism/disability which explicitly recognises the impact of structural and psycho-emotional barriers to inclusion would appear to have much to offer people with learning difficulties. Hall (2005) talked to people with learning difficulties living in Scotland who reported that whilst there were some cafés where their presence was welcomed, there were other establishments such as pubs where they were made to feel intimidated and unwelcome through unfriendly stares, hostile body language and hurtful comments. Consequently this group of people had a clear 'mental "map" of exclusionary and inclusionary spaces' (Hall, 2005, p. 109) which was shared with other people with learning difficulties living in the same town. This experience of being made to feel 'out of place' (Kitchin, 1998) is a good example of psycho-emotional disablism, showing the impact it had on the choices this group of people could make when deciding where to meet up socially.

Another important example of psycho-emotional disablism is that of disability hate crime and harassment – where someone who is perceived to be disabled is targeted for verbal or physical harassment, which unfortunately can escalate to injury or death. In 2009, 90 per cent of people with learning difficulties reported experiencing harassment or bullying (Sin et al., 2009), the highest percentage out of all impairment groups. Unfortunately, much of society views people with learning difficulties as being less human and having less emotional literacy than other people. This 'denial of psychological reality' (Murray, 2006, p. 38) about people with learning difficulties (and other disabled people) means that name calling and bullying is viewed as socially acceptable despite the very real harm done to self-esteem and personal safety. One example of this complacency is seen in the length of time it has taken to educate the police force about the need to record such incidents as examples of disability hate crime/harassment rather than 'anti-social behaviour' (EHRC, 2011).

The experience of disability hate crime and harassment can cause distress and anxiety, forcing people to change their choices about where they go in their local town in order to avoid perpetrators. Nonetheless, some people with learning difficulties are confident enough to challenge this form of psycho-emotional disablism. Here, Philip tells the interviewer (Ed) about the hassle he receives from an elderly neighbour:

Philip: I've got one neighbour, and every time I pass she shouts at me. One day I passed and I put the 'V sign' up.

Ed: Why does she shout at you?

Philip: Because of my disability. If she's got a problem, I said this to [another] neighbour and she said she's got an attitude problem, she's a bit dotty in her old age. I'll put you back in your place. As far as I'm concerned she can put her nose in the air, for all I care, but at the end of the day I'm 20 times taller than her.

(Hall, 2005, p. 111)

Philip knows that his neighbour shouts at him simply because he is disabled. Hall (2005) suggests that Philip deals with her ignorance by rendering his neighbour as the incompetent one – 'she's a bit dotty in her old age' – disrupting the connection between learning difficulties and competence. This could be seen as a form of resistance by Philip to being seen as inferior because he has a learning difficulty, although unfortunately, as Hall points out, he is achieving this gain by being ageist himself.

A disturbing example of *institutional* psycho-emotional disablism is revealed in the ongoing cases of institutional neglect and abuse exposed in care homes (such as Winterbourne View) and NHS assessment and treatment units (exemplified by the careless death of Connor Sparrowhawk). An evidence review looking at adult safeguarding and the social care workforce showed that after older people, adults with learning difficulties were the group most likely to experience abuse and neglect at the hands of care staff (Institute of Public Care, 2013). Disabled children experience more than three times the rates of abuse and neglect than do their non-disabled counterparts; children with learning difficulties (and those with communication impairments) carry a slightly increased risk compared to other impairment groups (Sullivan & Knutson, 2000). It has been suggested that sometimes 'diagnostic overshadowing' prevents health professionals from seeing psychological distress such as self-harming for what it is – an understandable response to trauma, harassment, abuse – rather than being assumed to be a 'natural' part of someone's impairment (Atkinson et al., 2014). I would argue that 'diagnostic overshadowing' is another example of institutional psycho-emotional disablism.

Finally I mentioned that internalised oppression is an important source of psycho-emotional disablism, one which is difficult to challenge because of the insidious way that stereotypes about disability are unconsciously incorporated into the psyche. Sinason describes clearly how the practice of amniocentesis can impact on the emotional well-being of people with learning difficulties:

> The deepest and most painful psychoanalytic theme that comes from long-term work is that learning disabled people can experience extreme annihilatory fear because it is hard (or impossible) to separate out the idea of amniocentesis or abortion of unborn learning disabled foetuses from a death wish towards learning disabled children and adults.
>
> (Sinason, 2002, p. 39)

Thus people with learning difficulties (and other disabled people) may feel acute anxiety about the value of their lives within society if this 'societal deathwish' has been internalised. However, this pain of societal rejection is often repressed and may only emerge after time in therapy, which clearly shows just how aware people with learning difficulties are of how others view them, contradicting the prejudice that such people lack the 'emotional intelligence' to be hurt in this way (Marks, 1999).

Conclusions

In the past the social model of disability has appeared to have less relevance for people with learning difficulties than other groups of disabled people because of the (unintended) focus on structural disablism. This chapter has shown that psycho-emotional disablism allows for the naming of forms of oppression which can have a devastating impact on the self-esteem and self-worth of people with learning difficulties. Therefore it is vitally important that professionals work systemically with someone with learning difficulties, remaining alert to the *potential* for both structural and psycho-emotional disablism in their lives, both past and present. My own research has shown the significant impact that caring, sensitive professionals can have on healing some of the damage done by psycho-emotional disablism, helping clients feel like valued human beings, worthy of being listened to and cared *about* (rather than *for*) (Reeve, 2008). Structural disablism can be difficult for an individual professional to personally fix, although it should always be challenged and solutions found where possible. However, because psycho-emotional disablism operates at the level of the interpersonal, the nature of the relationship between professional and person with learning difficulties is highly significant. Empathy – recognising that the person with learning difficulties is *'a real person I'm dealing with'* (Murray, 2006, p. 40, emphasis in original) with the same 'psychological reality' as everyone else – goes a long way towards facilitating an *enabling* rather than a *disabling* relationship between professional and person with learning difficulties.

Society has improved physical access for disabled people since the 1970s, forcing buildings to install lifts and ramps, providing accessible information for those disabled people that need it. However, negative attitudes and prejudices about disability, and in particular learning difficulties, are going to take a long time to improve because of the way that oppression tends to operate via:

> informal, often unnoticed and reflective speech, bodily reactions to others, conventional practices of everyday interactions and evaluation, aesthetic judgments and the jokes, images, and stereotypes pervading the mass media.

> (Young, 1990, p. 148)

In theory it is relatively straightforward to legislate to make buildings, services etc. accessible for disabled people, thereby removing structural disablism – people can see and touch these material barriers such as a flight of steps or confusing signs in a hospital. However, it is much harder to challenge the roots of prejudice and ableism which underpin psycho-emotional disablism, because the solutions rely on changes at the social and cultural level – changes which are harder to identify compared to a visible flight of steps or incomprehensible sign. Therefore, psycho-emotional disablism is not likely to disappear in the near future and so people with learning difficulties need support to deal with the distress caused by the name calling, bullying and harassment which, sadly, are a daily occurrence for this group of disabled people.

Box 3.1 Reflective questions on disability

- When was the last time you had a discussion with your clients about disablism and language? Or with your colleagues?

- In what ways might you be inadvertently disabling people with your words and actions?

- What forms of structural and psycho-emotional disablism do you notice in your working and/or personal life?

- To what extent does the service you work in take account of the ways in which people with learning difficulties experience and identify themselves? What possibilities might open up if this became more of a consideration?

- What practices might you and your organisation engage in that challenge psycho-emotional disablism and support recovery from its impact?

References

Atkinson, S., Dearden, D. & Dunne, C. (2014). The mental health needs of people with a learning disability. In S. Atkinson et al. (eds), *Intellectual Disability in Health and Social Care*, (pp. 380–409). Abingdon: Routledge.

Campbell, F.A.K. (2009). *Contours of Ableism: The Production of Disability and Abledness*. Basingstoke: Palgrave Macmillan.

Campbell, J. & Oliver, M. (1996). *Disability Politics: Understanding Our Past, Changing Our Future*. London: Routledge.

Chappell, A.L. (1997). From normalisation to where? In L. Barton & M. Oliver (eds), *Disability Studies: Past Present and Future*, (pp. 45–62). Leeds: The Disability Press.

Chappell, A.L., Goodley, D. & Lawthom, R. (2001). Making connections: The relevance of the social model of disability for people with learning difficulties. *British Journal of Learning Disabilities, 29*(2), 45–50.

Deal, M. (2003). Disabled people's attitudes toward other impairment groups: A hierarchy of impairments. *Disability & Society, 18*(7), 897–910.

EHRC. (2011). *Hidden in Plain Sight: Inquiry into Disability-Related Harassment.* London: Equality and Human Rights Commission.

Emerson, E. & Baines, S. (2011). Health inequalities and people with learning disabilities in the UK. *Tizard Learning Disability Review, 16*(1), 42–48.

Goodley, D. (2000). *Self-Advocacy in the Lives of People with Learning Difficulties.* Buckingham: Open University Press.

Hall, E. (2005). The entangled geographies of social exclusion/inclusion for people with learning disabilities. *Health & Place, 11*(2), 107–115.

Heslop, P. & Gordon, D. (2014). Trends in poverty and disadvantage among households with disabled people from 1999–2012: From exclusion to inclusion? *Journal of Poverty and Social Justice, 22*(3), 209–226.

Institute of Public Care (2013) *Evidence Review – Adult Safeguarding,* Skills for Care. https://ipc.brookes.ac.uk/publications/Evidence_Review_-_Adult_Safeguarding. pdf (accessed 10 December 2017).

Kitchin, R. (1998). 'Out of place', 'knowing one's place': Space, power and the exclusion of disabled people'. *Disability & Society, 13*(3), 343–356.

Marks, D. (1999). *Disability: Controversial Debates and Psychosocial Perspectives.* London: Routledge.

Murray, P. (2006). Being in school? Exclusion and the denial of psychological reality. In D. Goodley & R. Lawthom (eds), *Disability and Psychology: Critical Introductions and Reflections,* (pp. 34–41). London: Palgrave.

Oliver, M. (1990). *The Politics of Disablement.* London: Macmillan.

Reeve, D. (2002). Oppression within the counselling room. *Counselling and Psychotherapy Research, 2*(1), 11–19.

Reeve, D. (2008) *Negotiating Disability in Everyday Life: The Experience of Psycho-Emotional Disablism,* PhD Thesis, Lancaster University.

Reeve, D. (2014a). Counselling and disabled people: Help or hindrance? In J. Swain, S. French, C. Barnes & C. Thomas (eds), *Disabling Barriers – Enabling Environments,* 3rd edition (pp. 255–261). London: Sage.

Reeve, D. (2014b). Psycho-emotional disablism and internalised oppression. In J. Swain, S. French, C. Barnes & C. Thomas (eds), *Disabling Barriers – Enabling Environments,* 3rd edition (pp. 92–98). London: Sage.

Shakespeare, T. (2014). *Disability Rights and Wrongs Revisited,* 2nd edition. Abingdon: Routledge.

Sin, C.H., et al. (2009) *Disabled People's Experiences of Targeted Violence and Hostility (Research Report 21).* Manchester: Office for Public Management.

Sinason, V. (2002). Some reflections from twenty years of psychoanalytic work with children and adults with a learning disability. *Disability Studies Quarterly, 22*(3), 38–45.

Sullivan, P.M. & Knutson, J.F. (2000). Maltreatment and disabilities: A population-based epidemiological study. *Child Abuse & Neglect, 24*(10), 1257–1273.

Thomas, C. (2004). Developing the social relational in the social model of disability: A theoretical agenda. In C. Barnes & G. Mercer (eds), *Implementing the Social Model of Disability: Theory and Research*, (pp. 32–47). Leeds: The Disability Press.

Thomas, C. (2007). *Sociologies of Disability and Illness: Contested Ideas in Disability Studies and Medical Sociology*. Basingstoke: Palgrave Macmillan.

Tuffrey-Wijne, I. & Hollins, S. (2014). Preventing 'deaths by indifference': Identification of reasonable adjustments is key. *British Journal of Psychiatry*, 205(2), 86–87.

Young, I.M. (1990). *Justice and the Politics of Difference*. Princeton, NJ: Princeton University Press.

Young, S. (2014). *I'm not your inspiration, thank you very much*, [Internet], TEDxSydney. www.ted.com/talks/stella_young_i_m_not_your_inspiration_thank_you_very_much (accessed 15 December 2017).

4

Whose Story is it Anyway? A Narrative Approach to Working with People Affected by Learning Disabilities, Their Families and Networks

Sarah Coles and Helen Ellis-Caird

Accessible summary

- There are many stories told in society about how people affected by learning disabilities live their lives and manage difficulties.

- These stories influence the ways professionals may interact with people.

- We should ask people what their own life stories are.

- The chapter talks about the background theory to narratives and telling our stories.

- We talk about increasing the opportunity for people with learning disabilities to story their lives, and about sharing stories with others.

We are clinical psychologists who since qualifying have been interested in working in ways that draw on our clients' strengths, values and resources. There are many stories told in society about how people affected by learning disabilities live their lives and manage difficulties, for example the idea that their learning disability is an explanation for any difficulty they encounter rather than a normal part of life. Having both worked with people affected by learning disability we have witnessed the totalising effect of a 'learning disability' diagnosis on people's lives, leaving little room for other stories to be told and heard. We have found that we can get drawn into these descriptions, for example noticing the diagnosis before the person, and the problem before understanding a life story. The 'learning disability' can become an

explanation for everything; indeed, our services would not work with someone without a learning disability. Particularly with the pressure of being in
a busy NHS team, we have noticed how we and other professionals can be
organised by these discourses into narrow ways of responding to our clients'
problems. This limits the resources that we have to impact change, and
diminishes the opportunity for people affected by learning disabilities to story
their own lives.

We have been drawn to narrative ideas as a way of countering these discourses, reconnecting with our curiosity and opening up possibilities for
change. This feels like a more ethical way of working and fits with our values of
equality, fairness, justice and respect. It enables us to give voice to those in our
society who are often marginalised and discriminated against.

Underpinning narrative theory

Narrative therapy is built on a rich bed of ideas drawn from postmodern and
post-structuralist philosophy, literary theory and anthropology. We cannot begin
to do justice to these roots here, so will focus in on just one important figure
in the development of narrative therapy: Michel Foucault, a French philosopher,
historian of ideas, social theorist, and literary critic.

Foucault's (1975) ideas are central to the development of narrative
therapy. He proposed that society is structured by a number of dominant
narratives or discourses which inform how we think about ourselves and
how we interact with each other. These dominant narratives in society shape
our opinions and action, thus limiting our ways of viewing and interpreting
actions (Dallos & Draper, 2010). Throughout history dominant groups have
asserted their authority over language though control of the production
of knowledge, of what is published and of access to education (Hare-
Mustin & Marecek, 1990). This means that dominant discourses which are
available to story our lives are largely shaped by the powerful in society. It
therefore makes sense that for less powerful groups, like those with learning
disabilities, who have limited access to the use of language and means of
producing knowledge, the opportunity to tell their own story is severely
constrained.

Michael White, the founder of narrative therapy, was greatly influenced by
Foucault's thinking, and recognised the central importance of the stories we
tell to make sense of our experiences. When the stories we tell are limited or
are narrowly focused by dominant discourse, a non-preferred account of our
lives can be all we have to tell. White referred to these as 'problem-saturated'
stories which are often told and retold, growing stronger and more central,
meaning that 'shy' stories which may chronicle our strengths and values can
be forgotten and left untold. In a learning disabilities context, the incidence

of 'problem-saturated' stories abounds. Limited speech to express oneself and limited memory capacity may undermine the ability of a person to tell their own stories, and to form and maintain a preferred coherent story about their life (Coles et al., 2012). In these circumstances, thick paper files full of the opinions and perspectives of those in a position of relative power can take on undue influence.

Box 4.1 Storytelling exercise

It can be hard to recognise the power that stories have to narrate our lives. In the exercise which follows we're asking you to consider what it's like to tell different stories about your own life, and how these tellings can impact the way we feel about and see ourselves. When engaging in the exercise, ensure you choose stories that feel safe for you to tell.

- Working in pairs, tell a story about a time you found difficult at school and a story about a time you felt good at school.

- Which story did you prefer?

- What was the effect on you emotionally of telling these different stories?

- What was the effect on the listener of both stories?

- What impact would telling more of each kind of story have on how you see yourself and your actions?

In moving away from 'professionalised' and what they called 'experience distant' depictions of people's lives, White and Epston (1990) championed an alternative way to work in therapy and for professionals to use in wider community roles. In narrative work, the person is centred as the expert in their own life, with the role of the therapist being to create opportunities for 're-authoring' practices, supporting the uncovering of 'preferred' stories, which tell of the skills, competencies, beliefs, values, commitments and abilities that the person has available to them. Through the thickening and enriching of these stories, the potentially pathologising and limiting influence of problem-saturated stories can be lessened.

Key concepts

We take these narrative ideas as the foundation from which we try to approach our work. Next we would like to share with you some of our 'go to' clinical practices, which influence all aspects of our work, that are drawn from these foundations.

Box 4.2 Our clinical practice toolkit

Deconstruction and positioning: throughout the client referral and assessment process, we try and notice the assumptions present in the way referrals are conceptualised and spoken about.

Externalising: we ensure that we think of problems as separate to people in the way we use language; for example we talk of 'the anxiety' not 'your anxiety'.

Curiosity: we attempt to remain curious rather than making assumptions, for example about the impact and effects of the problem on the person's life and those around them.

Preferred stories: we ensure that we hear the client's preferred stories and stories not affected by the problem, and take time to amplify them.

Documenting: ethically, we feel that documenting these new and less problem-focused stories is important because it can counter stories of people's lives that are often contained in health records.

Spreading the news: we may invite others to hear these new stories, or to think about how these ideas can be included within support plans. We also think carefully about the ending of client work, ensuring the end is marked using certificates, letters and *definitional ceremonies* to acknowledge and celebrate the work.

Putting these ideas into practice – A reflective case study

Mark, a 40-year-old white British man, was referred to a multidisciplinary team in rural England. There were concerns regarding vulnerability in managing finances (money spent gambling) and also his ability to self-care. He was living in his family home but his parents had both died and his brother had recently moved away. The team wondered if he was able to live alone or if he should move to supported living. He was diagnosed with a mild learning disability.

The initial referral into the team was made by a social worker, who wanted a psychologist to conduct an assessment of Mark's capacity in relation to his ability to manage his finances and live alone. An intervention for his gambling habit was also requested.

Helen: Looking back, it seems that the referral into the service was focused on what Mark was unable to do and the ensuing multidisciplinary team (MDT) conversation perpetuated a story of risk, vulnerability and inability. By the end of the conversation, I remember that it seemed there was no option but to move Mark to a more supported setting to protect him. On reflection, it felt like Mark's voice was lost in this discussion in relation to his view of his difficulties, and also his strengths, values and hopes for his own life. This was uncomfortable for me and also for the other members of the MDT who had entered their careers to champion the rights of people affected by disability, yet the stories of protection and risk management prevailed. Some of the narrative ideas we introduced above could have created possibilities for different stories. It seems that as a team we lost our curiosity, which meant that the context for the referral and the assumptions in it were left unquestioned. If the MDT discussion had been informed by narrative ideas of *'deconstruction and positioning'* we could have asked questions within this conversation such as:

➢ *Who else would share these ideas?*

➢ *Who might think differently?*

➢ *What else is going on for this person?*

➢ *Why the referral now? What has changed?*

➢ *What are the strengths and values this person might have?*

➢ *What is Mark's relationship to the problem?*

➢ *What is the social worker's relationship to the problem?*

➢ *What social practices might be contributing to this problem?*

➢ *What other stories are there about Mark?*

This may have allowed a more complex picture of Mark to emerge which may have opened up possibilities for different actions more quickly. Instead, Mark was, referred to me for individual therapy to reduce the gambling behaviour and for a capacity assessment.

Meeting Mark face to face, I was struck by how little I knew about him beyond the narrow questions of risk and capacity discussed in the MDT. Holding in mind narrative ideas around *curiosity* and *deconstruction*, I started to talk with him about gambling using the narratively informed questions below:

➢ *What is the problem?*

➢ *When did it start? Has it always been a problem? When did it change?*

➢ *Who else would notice the problem?*

➢ *Who are its friends? Who are its supporters?*

➤ *When is the problem bigger and smaller?*

➤ *Do you think the problem is good or bad?*

➤ *What are the problem's effects and plans for your life?*

Mark was able to explain that gambling had been a part of his life since he was a child, when his dad used to take him to the horse races. It was something he and his brother used to do together, going weekly to the same betting shop to place a bet. Mark told me that he had started going more often after his brother moved out. He said the betting shop was a place where everybody knew him and welcomed him, and knew his father before him. Mark said it was a place he felt safe and warm, and could have a cheap meal. This contrasted to his own home, where he was now living alone, without heating and without his brother who was always the one who had done the cooking. For Mark, then, it quickly emerged that gambling in itself was not the problem; it was in fact a way of staying connected with a sense of family and community. The thing that was problematic for Mark was a sense of loneliness and isolation since his parents had died and his brother had left, which had resulted in the frequency of gambling increasing. Mark was aware that this was a problem and that he didn't have enough money to go every day, but the loneliness he felt at home meant that he kept going back.

*Our focus shifted to talk in more detail about Mark's perception of the current problem, which revolved around a sense of loneliness and unhappiness being home alone. Mark spoke of never really having friends and feeling that people don't like him and think he's weird. He told me he'd always felt a bit like this and that since his parents had died and his brother had left, he really had no one to talk to which made him very sad. There was something very definite and fixed in the way Mark was talking, as if loneliness was very much a part of who he was. I therefore decided to use the narrative idea of **externalising**, using words and drawing to get some space between Mark and loneliness. The kinds of questions I used to support this included:*

➤ *If you could draw loneliness, what do you think it would look like?*

➤ *What colours might it be? Would it be a dark or light colour?*

➤ *How big might loneliness be?*

➤ *Would it have smooth edges or spiky edges?*

➤ *What would be a good name for this picture?*

Mark drew a picture of himself, and drew a bubble around himself with jagged edges. He called the bubble the 'stay away bubble' and said that it makes him feel sad, and all by himself. He explained that when the bubble surrounded him, he feels like no one likes him or wants him around and it makes it hard for him to think of anything to say. He told me that the 'stay away bubble' plans for Mark to always be alone and not to have a good life. Mark spoke of going to the betting shop as a time when the bubble lifted a little, as it was a place where he and his family were known, people said 'Hello' to him, and where he could talk about horses, a subject he knows lots about.

It seemed that going to the betting shop was actually an example of an exception to what was otherwise quite a problem-saturated story, in which the 'stay away bubble' kept Mark alone and isolated. Remaining curious, I explored for further times in which the cloud lifted, and Mark spoke more about going out and about with his father, walking the family dog, going to the shops. Mark told me his father would always say 'Hello' to people they met, and that times with him were very happy, and the 'stay away bubble' would lift.

Our work continued with us exploring further Mark's relationship with his father using narrative techniques of **re-membering** to help reconnect Mark with some of the values that he shared with his father, and open up more **preferred stories**. This included the importance of family to both him and his dad, and Mark's wish to stay close to his memories of his parents, but also the importance of being a part of a community and knowing people in his area.

These stories opened up very different possibilities of ways of working with Mark to expand the ways in which he could lift up the 'stay away bubble' without spending as much money on gambling. Mark and I agreed that he start work with the team's occupational therapist (OT) to explore ways of **thickening stories** of being close to his family and honouring different family traditions (alongside gambling), for example by cleaning the house, or learning to cook his traditional family meals. These were actions that were in line with values (being close to his family and remembering them) and his hopes for feeling more comfortable in his home. Mark was also introduced to a support worker. In line with the importance Mark placed on being a part of the community, the support worker went with Mark to check out local community groups, and Mark began to attend a local day centre for people with learning disabilities. The support worker also aided Mark to get his heating repaired and carry out a weekly shop, actions which increased his comfort at home and his confidence to shop beyond the local bookmakers.

Mark's gambling decreased and his community network grew stronger, he began attending the day centre once a week, and, with support from the OT and support worker, learnt a number of basic recipes that he was proud to cook for himself. The 'stay away bubble' was still there at times for Mark, but he described it as lighter and said that he could now pop it when he needed to.

As Mark and I approached the end of our narrative therapy work, our thoughts turned to how to document and share stories with others. In narrative language this is called *spreading the news*. Our intention was to share the *new preferred stories* that had emerged from our conversations. We spent some time thinking about how Mark would like these ideas shared and who with, and who could support him in keeping going with his new activities. Mark decided that he would like his brother, support worker and the social worker to come to a final meeting to take part in an '*Outside Witnessing Ceremony*'. This was a chance for Mark to talk about what was important to him, and was also about how knowing more people were helping to lift the 'stay away bubble'. He spoke about how important family was to him and staying close to the memory of his mum and dad by keeping his house warm and cooking for himself. Through outside witnessing questions, his brother, support worker and social worker were able to amplify and give back to Mark this *thickened story*, and demonstrate its value to them and their own lives.

As a team we were careful to write Mark a letter *documenting* all the stories which had emerged which provided a contrast to the initial referral letter – an extract of this second letter is reproduced below:

Dear Mark,

... we talked about your Dad. You told me that he was a very nice man who always wore a hat. You liked to go for walks together with your dogs. These were good times because the stay away bubble would lift, and you and your Dad would say hello to people that you met. Your Dad liked to know everyone and this is something that you like too.

You've been meeting with XX and have got to know some of the people who work in the shops by XX and you've also started going to the XX Centre. This has felt really good, it makes you think of your Dad because now people know you and say hello.

Looking back on this work, it seems that the gambling was one of many stories to be told about Mark's life, his hobbies and hopes. The referral took one view and made this a dominant story – of a vulnerable man with a serious gambling habit. Through the use of a narrative approach we discovered a more nuanced story and, with support from the OT and support worker, we were able to give Mark the ability to thicken and strengthen alternative stories aligned with his values and hopes for the future. We hope that this case study demonstrates some of the ways that narrative approaches can be used by different members of an MDT to enable us to be more curious about our work, to notice our assumptions, to separate the person from the problem and to open up possibilities for change.

Reflection on the impact of narrative ideas on our ways of working

Narrative ideas allow us to think transparently about the way society and policy influence the assumptions we might make about disability. It highlights the ways in which the structure of organisations (referral systems etc.) influence how we are invited into people's lives, and how once we are there we have obligations, duties and responsibilities that encourage us to take particular positions (e.g. protectionism). We have found that this approach enables us to question ideas and assumptions that we hold. It makes us question our inherent beliefs about what we are being invited to do in our jobs within a learning disability team. It helps us reflect on our practice through questions like:

> *Is this a helpful thing to be doing for the person who has been referred to us?*

> *What would we be saying if learning disability wasn't around?*

> *What are the preferred stories the person might want to tell about their life?*

> *Are my views about this, combined with the power I have as part of my role, too dominant?*

We also find this a positive way of working as we are able not only to look at problems and limitations but to look at what the person can do and wants to do. Where can this person feel a sense of agency? How do they want to change and make things different? This can be hard when stories of protectionism and safety are often at the front of professionals' minds, but if we stay mindful of this pull then there are usually places where the person can begin to grow these different ways of being, allowing positive risk taking. It is also a respectful way of working as it places the person at the centre of the storytelling about their lives in a way that doesn't always happen. It amplifies the person's voice about the kind of world they want to live in.

Conclusion

In summary, we have found the narrative approach to be beneficial when working in systems that include learning disability, in a number of ways: thinking about wider social discourses and assumptions; creating different types of conversations that do not centre on deficits; and creating a sense of agency for the person in their own life. This way of working, in turn, is inspiring and creative, which allows us to remain joyful in our work.

Box 4.3 Common questions/dilemmas when using a narrative approach

There are a number of common concerns that people new to this way of thinking have raised with us in teaching and supervision, and we thought we would try to address these questions here.

If you externalise a problem, for example anger, do you not run the risk of reducing the person's sense of responsibility for the impact of anger on others, and potentially their ability to change their behaviour?

This is a good question and people often have similar concerns relating to issues of violence and power. The intention of externalising is to reduce the impact of 'totalization' of the label (White, 1986); that is, the person is not an angry person but the anger has influence over the person's life. Externalising conversations can make it possible for people to take more responsibility and to have more of a sense of agency about how to make changes in their life. Externalising is not about separating the person from the actions or the impact on others of their behaviour. Indeed, externalising carefully details all of the effects and influence the anger might have, as well as where these ideas might have come from, and what discourses in society might maintain anger's influence, for example discourses of gender or power. It is also, of course, the therapist's responsibility to consider the safety of others with regard to issues of anger, power and accountability and to ensure these conversations are bought into the therapy room. Our belief is that externalising means that a person can take a different position to their problem; this can enable them to begin to think differently about it, which in turn opens up possibility for change.

If you resist the discourses of risk and protectionism, are you not at risk yourself of not acting responsibly or not complying with the obligations, roles and responsibilities inherent in your work?

Another good question. In our view, this way of working allows increased transparency about the discourses which might be influencing our ideas of our work roles. For example, the strong discourse around our job being to 'risk manage' might make us take up a protectionist position focused on limitations and deficits, whereas noticing shy stories about strengths and abilities might make us more likely to encourage positive risk taking. This is not an either/or position, but by taking a more curious perspective we can better notice these discourses and question our allegiance to them. This is in no way counter to the responsibilities and accountability of members of the MDT to consider the safety of our clients and to comply with our organisations' structures (risk assessment), as well as our obligations to act in ethical and professional ways (though at times these may need questioning). On the contrary, narrative ideas encourage us to think critically about our values and responsibilities rather than following well-trodden paths of taken-for-granted discourses.

▶

◄ ⏐

I'm concerned that drawing with people affected by learning disabilities might be considered inappropriate?

In the 1970s, Wolfensberger introduced the normalisation principle, in which the importance of people with learning disabilities living 'ordinary' lives was stressed. This was pivotal policy at a time when many with learning disabilities were confined to institutions, and it formed the legal basis for affirming rights to education, work, and community living. As part of this, the importance of considering a person's chronological age was stressed, as a counter to the dehumanising and infantilising treatment of past ages. In our opinion, this was an incredibly progressive movement within its historical context, but viewed in today's context can risk a focus on what is 'appropriate' for a person, rather than what the person likes, or what makes sense to a person. For us, communicating with a person affected by learning disability in a way that makes sense to them is respectful and appropriate, in a way that talking to someone using language that they do not understand is not. If a person with a learning disability likes to draw, and if this can enhance communication, then drawing is appropriate. If they do not like drawing and it does not facilitate communication, then it is not appropriate. We therefore see this as a decision made with the individual rather than as a blanket decision influenced by theoretical and historical contexts.

References

Coles, S., Caird, H. & Rikberg Smyly, S. (2012). Remember my voice. *Clinical Psychology & People with Learning Disabilities*, 10(2), 44–48.

Dallos, R. & Draper, R. (2010). *An Introduction to Family Therapy: Systemic Theory and Practice*. New York: Open University Press.

Foucault, M. (1975) *The Archaeology of Knowledge*. London: Tavistock.

Hare-Mustin, R. & Marecek, J. (1990). *Making a Difference: Psychology and the Construction of Gender*. New Haven, CT: Yale University Press.

White, M. (1986). Negative explanation, restraint, and double description: A template for family therapy. *Family Process*, 25, 169–184.

White, M. & Epston, D. (1990). *Narrative Means to Therapeutic Ends*. New York: WW Norton.

Wolfensberger, W. (1998). *A Brief Introduction to Social Role Valorization: A High-order Concept for Addressing the Plight of Societally Devalued People, and for Structuring Human Services*, 3rd edition. Syracuse, NY: Training Institute for Human Service Planning, Leadership and Change Agentry (Syracuse University).

5

Beginning to Work Systemically: Working with Referrals

Lorna Robbins

Accessible summary

- Before we start working with someone we should think about these questions:
  - what have we been asked to do?
  - who has asked us?
  - why have they asked us?
  - why are they asking now?
  - who is it important for us to talk to?
- When we use systemic ideas it can change the way that we work with people.
- When we use systemic ideas it can change the ways that teams work together.

When thinking about how to use systemic ideas in our practice, an obvious starting point is the first point of contact, that is, the referral. This chapter is interested in exploring the following practice-based considerations:

What is the context of the referral and how might we know if this referral is suitable for a systemic approach?

How might systemic ideas shape the referral and triage process, and how might we share these ideas with colleagues in the team?

What are the systemic ideas/concepts/practices that can be employed when one starts working with a referral?

What does a systemic approach suggest about how to understand and respond to referrals?

Reflections from the South West Systemic Learning
Disability Special Interest Group.

Throughout each section there will be illustrations of the sorts of questions we might ask about a referral.

People with learning disabilities' problems are rarely theirs alone, or held in isolation, thus although the referral will very often describe *the problem* in relation to a specific person, at the point of referral it is helpful to be open minded about the way *the problem* is conceptualised. With the advent of popular and powerful schools of thought such as cognitive behavioural therapy (see Kushlick et al., 1997; Sturmey, 2004; Hwang & Kearney, 2013; Idusohan-Moizer et al., 2015) and more recently the revival of behavioural interventions in the form of positive behaviour support (see Allen et al., 2005; Gore et al., 2013; Hassiotis, 2014; NICE, 2015) there is a tendency to focus on the individual and the problem located in or around the individual, rather than having a wider focus that is relational and putting the problem into the context of the system around it. On the other hand, a balance must be maintained to ensure the perspective and voice of the person with learning disability is properly included.

What is the context of the referral and how might we know if this referral is suitable for a systemic approach?

The context of where we work will shape the referrals we receive and how we think about responding to them. Over recent years, services have changed considerably, and so the context of those sending, and of those receiving, referrals is likely to be different and with specific contextual markers depending on where you are based.

Professional and agency context

The Community Team for Adults with Learning Disabilities (CTALD) in which I work as a clinical psychologist and systemic therapist has in recent years separated from being co-located with the local authority, and now sits more firmly within the NHS and local mental health provision, relabelled a Learning Disabilities Specialist Health Service. Such separations can cause tensions between services with how to work together and ensure we are thinking about a referral or presenting need in a holistic or joined-up way. Arguably this is the very reason that a systemic approach remains such an important component of truly integrative, person-centred but holistic care. Locally another contextual marker, and perhaps a change in the language used, is a focus on and attention to risk, assessing it and managing it effectively. Whilst the language and processes around risk might sometimes feel mechanistic, this is an area where systemic ideas and approaches help us to be thoughtful and make sense together of these complex dynamics, ensuring everyone is kept safe whilst also developing opportunities for those involved to move towards improved quality of life and relationships with others.

There will be those referrals that seem to clearly fit with a systemic approach and where the referrer is requesting a systemic intervention. These might include referrals for family therapy, couple work, or relational/systemic individual therapy. How able your referrers are to request or name a type of intervention may be influenced by their training, experience, beliefs, knowledge of different models of therapy, and expectations about what different types of intervention may offer. We have found that it is helpful to send out information leaflets (including accessible ones, see Table 5.1) so potential referrers are more aware of what is available and how it might be helpful to their client (i.e. that we can see groups of people living together, people attending with their network of support, adults with their parents). We have also found meeting face to face to discuss what a systemic intervention might look like helps referrers to make more appropriate referrals, and helps clients and their network of support feel more able to give informed consent to the therapeutic process; in addition, any concerns or barriers to engagement can be addressed. The experience of co-construction or being part of a collaborative process is thus put into practice from the point of referral.

Other types of referral are less obviously systemic ones, for example for behaviour that challenges or consultation with a care provider, where the team are likely to look to positive behaviour support or similar approaches. In my service we have a daily 'Single Point of Access' (SPA) conference call where a representative from each professional group in the multidisciplinary team (MDT) discusses each referral and considers who is best to triage, determine urgency, and decide which care pathway the referral relates to. I am sure other services have a variation on this theme; whether a group of practitioners or an individual, we are all trying to make sense of what is being requested, who is best placed to help and the urgency of the work. Again, much like other services, we have developed NICE guidance-informed MDT care pathways to help practitioners offer a consistent and best-practice process across

Table 5.1   Part of the information leaflet we use for the systemic therapy clinic, to explain our use of the reflecting team approach

	The therapists work as a team.		In another room, there will be up to 4 other therapists. They will watch and listen. They are thinking about new ideas and things that might help.
	You will be in a room with a therapist and your family/ network of support.		After about 40 minutes the other therapists will come into the room and talk together. They will share their ideas with you and the family/network of support.
	The therapist will listen and talk with you all.		The therapists can help us have more ideas, understand your difficulties better, and also notice things that are helping things to improve.

the county. These include eligibility, dementia, behaviour that challenges and mental health pathways. Although our behaviour that challenges pathway follows NICE guidance (NICE 2016, 2017) which largely endorses a positive behaviour support approach, we endeavour to incorporate a systemic stance, situating the difficulties as relational, being attentive to the context around the person, and asking questions in a way that is congruent with a systemic approach. Practitioners in the team think about the way in which questions are asked or bring in the idea of multiple lenses to thicken the quality and robustness of the assessment and subsequent interventions (see Table 5.1).

From the point of referral and the beginning of the client's journey with our service, the importance of having a systemic lens to view the referral, ask questions about it and influence how we think it might be most appropriately taken forward is crucial. Due to capacity and demand pressures I am aware that in other services psychological practitioners or systemic therapists might not be included in the first point of contact discussions as their time is viewed as better spent in direct clinical work. However, the opportunity to view referrals through a systemic lens from the very beginning of a client's journey seems to be a good use of time, ensuring that the team response reflects some of the systemic values and approaches to intervening in difficulties (e.g. curiosity, a relational focus to difficulties, inclusion of multiple perspectives, attention to power, difference and culture, attention to the language used about and by a person). Like the rest of us, people with learning disabilities' problems do not exist in isolation and do not reside in any one individual, but rather sit within a complex network of interactions with others around them.

Box 5.1 How do I know if a systemic approach is appropriate?

Reflections to help you consider the suitability and/or utility of a systemic approach:

Triage stage –

- *What are the views of others?*

- *How can we include others' perspectives as part of the work?*

- *Does anyone have a different view?*

- *Who might we need to talk to in order to get a wider range of ideas about the problem?*

- *How can we pay attention to and open up space for other stories about the person/relationships/situation?*

- *Drawing on White's (1995) concept that our lives are multi-storied, how can we be attentive to other stories about the person?*

- *How can we encourage different ideas to be brought in at the triage stage to enable a shift away from pervasive negative accounts and stories of hopelessness?*

- *How can we use curiosity to learn how certain events may be connected, and what sense the person has made of this experience? Can we get information to sequence events across time? What meaning has the person, family, carers, referrer attached to these experiences, and what is the meaning they give to events that would allow connection to an alternative story?*

▶

- *Attention to unique outcomes. How can we obtain information about when the problem isn't around? What can we learn from this? As part of the triage process how can we bring in space for 'hope' – invite initial thoughts that there might be something different/a different future without the problem?*

- *Being sensitive to the use of language. What words would we use to talk about the problem, situation around the person, relationships and so on? What would help shift the dialogue in a positive direction? What is the meaning of certain language for those involved?*

How might systemic ideas shape the referral and triage process, and how might we share these ideas with colleagues in the team?

As part of our triage process we will consider how to get started, and how change might be introduced and subsequently maintained. Initially we are trying to understand the problem. At both SPA and then triage, we explore an appreciation of what each person has been experiencing (the referrer, the client and those in their network of support), and consider the person and the referrer's experience of the problem (how does the problem affect their lives and relationships?). As part of this process we aim to assist the referrer to describe the problem or concern. Initially they may recount the concerns in a way that has been stated many times, what White would call a 'thin description' (1995). So as part of the triaging and making-sense process we encourage a more relational account that considers the effects of the problem on people's lives. This includes the emotional, behavioural, physical, and interactional effects, and the meaning being made about the problem by those involved. Drawing further on narrative ideas (White, 1995) we might ask questions along the lines of:

Is the person (are you) experiencing any health concerns which might be related to the problem (e.g. anxiety/depression/physical illness) and what is the impact of these on their (your) life?

Are there factors in the person's home/placement setting that contribute to the current situation?

Have there been staffing or other changes that might have had an impact on the lives of the residents/relationships in the setting?

When did you first notice this being a problem? Who finds it most difficult? Is there anyone who seems to manage the problem better?

Is the problem affecting anything else in the situation/your life which you haven't mentioned? Can you tell me more about it?

What do other people think, say or do about the problem? What difference does that make? How do you talk about it together?

Where did these ideas come from? Have you ever come across different ways of thinking about this?

Are there ideas from the media, national guidance documents and so on that influence the way the problem is thought about/influence your thoughts about the placement/care provision?

Are there things you have learnt from similar situations that would be helpful here? Would these things be similar or different for someone without an intellectual disability? If so, in what way? What sense do you make of that? Can we draw on ideas from other life-stage transitions that might be useful here?

These types of question encourage a wider perspective, and warm the context for starting to think differently about a 'problem' that people have become concerned about or stuck over how to resolve.

A second aspect of responding to the referral is creating a context for a new way of thinking about the problem, where it is not considered intrinsic to any one person but something that is between people. This can be a real and difficult shift in the way of thinking about and talking about a problem. Referrals are often framed or described as internalised problems (i.e. held within one person), and as a consequence we are naturally drawn to internalising conversations (focusing on an individual and talking as if the problem is within them). To bring systemic ideas into our practice we might try to shift from a position of 'Joe Bloggs is the problem; he needs to change' to 'How is the problem affecting Joe's life and his relationships? How is the problem impacting on the referrer/ people around Joe?'. An example might be of a referral for someone with challenging 'attention seeking' behaviour, and a request to, in effect, fix them, possibly by using medication or advice to 'manage their behaviour'. A new way of thinking about the problem might be to explore relationships between people, the context or environment around the problem, and develop shared understandings about how we all might want to interact or gain attention/attachments with others and share difficult feelings, and ways that the person could do this without having to resort to angry outbursts.

What are the systemic ideas/concepts/practices that are employed when one starts working with a referral?

Systemic ideas and theories are broad and have evolved significantly over time. However, some concepts remain core foundations for a comprehensive triage of a referral. Drawing on ideas from Burnham (1986) and Halliday and Robbins (2006), it would be helpful to consider the following when working with a referral.

> ➤ A systems focus. Systemic practitioners seek to look beyond the individual and see the wider system as the 'client'. They aim to identify the meaning and function of a presenting problem within the context of the system in which it has developed. This makes it easier to consider how to facilitate meaningful change. Therefore one would want to explore whether there are any sequences or themes in the individual, family or systems history. Are there any repetitive behavioural patterns or enduring beliefs that are interconnected in the person's system of support? For example, there might be a family story that values being 'strong, tough, speaking your mind, standing up for yourself'. For the family member with the intellectual disability, if this is enacted through aggression rather than assertive talk, this is likely to become a problem. Exploring the meaning behind such beliefs and finding other ways of feeling 'strong' and 'standing up for yourself' might be helpful not just to the person with the intellectual disability but to all those in the system. Another example would be around times of transition. What ideas do the person with the intellectual disability, family members and others in the system have about growing up, leaving home and becoming independent? Where did these beliefs originate from; what influences them; which are shared ideas; and where do ideas, hopes and expectations differ?

> ➤ Problems are seen in the context of relationships, rather than located within a single individual. Practitioners would therefore want to consider relationship styles and patterns, and the development of rules, stories or ways of being between the people involved. How might these be contributing to the difficulty? How might these offer avenues for facilitating change?

> ➤ Problems are also seen in a wider context of the person's situation or placement. Therefore we would be curious to know more about this: what informs these ideas and what do they add to the understanding of the problem? What are the environmental circumstances (size of accommodation, availability of meaningful activities, choice of friendships); what

are the cultural factors that we need to take into account? In exploring relationship patterns, we should pay attention to concepts such as the connectedness, relational processes and communication styles of those involved.

➤ Using collaborative processes, we would be looking to develop shared goals and make the intervention bespoke to the client needs, for example by altering the pace of the sessions and the type of language employed, and using creativity to allow everyone to contribute to the process.

➤ Problems can become more apparent or emerge at a time of transition. Carter and McGoldrick's *Family Life Cycle* (1980) resonates when used in the context of learning disabilities, providing a basis for conversations about change, normative expectations, differences and the potential impact these might have. In slightly different presentations, in our work we often pick up on a theme of adults with a learning disability seeking appropriate independence but parents treating them as if they were still a child, being overly protective of them compared to other siblings. Although the intentions are usually to be caring, the outcome is often a restriction of community access and of opportunities to have a job or relationships or to leave home. Very often frustrations struggle to get communicated verbally, so this tension gets acted out between family members, often serving to concern the parents further about their child's ability to live independently, and so a 'stuckness' prevents smooth transitioning.

➤ A systemic approach would be curious about times when problems are less evident, what is making a positive difference and what we can learn from this. Practitioners would be attentive to noticing stories of resources in the system, stability, and the capacity to change within the system.

➤ Practitioners largely adopt a non-expert position and draw on local knowledge from those joining in the process. Rather than being an expert-led directive process, the approach is reflective both in terms of style of conversation, and by use of methods such as a reflecting team.

Practice considerations (including, collaborating, adjusting, intervening, engaging and exploring)

➤ *Including*: who is the 'customer', i.e. the person who most wants to effect change? What led the referrer to make the referral now? Who else is aware of the referral and what is their view? What is/might be the view of the referred person(s) about the problem? How can we involve the relevant people, and what is the most appropriate way to do this?

➤ *Collaborating*: what are the expectations of all involved; which of these are shared; are there ideas around shared goals; how might we negotiate the frame of the work; how might we decide the type of intervention or model choice (family therapy, individual therapy, a systemic consultation to the network of support)? In my work this decision-making process consists of my having conversations with those involved to make sense of where the focus of the work is most likely to be helpful; what has been tried before and how this effected change; whether the person with the intellectual disability has capacity to understand and be involved in the change process; or whether any work is in their best interests. For example, are the difficulties located within the staff team dynamics and is work best undertaken at this level, or is the difficulty between the person with the learning disability and those close to them, and can they all be invited to join a talking therapy approach?

➤ *Adjusting*: how to include everyone's voice/views; how we might use creative approaches to gathering information (pictures, drawing, sand tray); what style of questions will open up a dialogue between us; the language used and what impact this might have on the way the problem is constructed between those involved; what impact this has on the referred person.

➤ *Intervening using an ability discourse*: by their very nature, referrals are usually problem focused and often full of accounts related to the influence of disability on the person's life and those around them. By being curious about strengths, resources, values and hopes in the system, we have found we are more able to move to a position of feeling ready for change and thinking about solutions.

➤ *Engaging*: where there is a history of difficulty with connecting with services, what might we need to know about that; what are the stories around change processes; what is the current relationship; and how might we do things differently? We can ensure supervision/reflective processes are in place as part of good practice, but particularly draw on them if or when the work gets stuck. As a team it can be helpful to consider what would define the work as a success or failure. Would this relate to unmet goals, therapeutic challenges, agency conflicts, record keeping, skills required, practitioner relationship to the problem/relationships around the problem, the timing of the work, pace of the work, or disagreements over the 'problem', its causes, and/or ways to alter the situation?

➤ *Exploring conversations*: I have found questions that deconstruct the problem to be useful (adapted from White, 1989, pp. 37–46, cited in Payne, 2000):

How did you get yourself ready to take this step?

Would you describe to me the circumstances surrounding this referral?

Did anyone else contribute to this and if so in what way? If they were part of this discussion is there anything else that they might add?

What would the referred person(s) say if they were listening? What leads you to think that might be their view?

What do you/the staff team/carers believe to be important in the referred person's life? What do you think it might say about your hopes/values as a staff team?

What has been helpful in the past? How have they/you coped with challenging times previously that might be useful to consider now?

During our discussion I have been struck by your commitment to meeting the referred person's needs. Where does this commitment come from? How does it get supported by your organisation? Is there anything further that would help to support you and the wider team?

Working with people with learning disabilities, their care teams, families and wider networks of support, I have tended to take the gist of Michael White's questions and simplify them and make them more concrete, as this seems to make them more accessible whilst still helping us to think about the problem or situation from a new angle. Altering the types of question used so that there is a shift to less familiar ways of thinking can need to be negotiated (in systemic conversations this is often referred to as 'warming the context', that is gently preparing for a conversation or question); it can help if these questions are not too different initially, so that people can adapt their narratives and ways of talking about/thinking about and making sense of the difficulties.

What does a systemic approach suggest about how to understand and respond to referrals? Reflections from the South West Systemic Learning Disability Special Interest Group

The following extracts from a reflecting discussion illustrate some potential dilemmas and ways forward when beginning to work systemically with referrals. Practitioners work in NHS community learning disability teams (CLDTs) across the south west, and include those from psychology, nursing and academic backgrounds.

Taking an ethical position

We need to encourage others to remember that in effect the person being referred is already a client, and so to hold a philosophy or position that part of the referral process is to think in ways that are helpful to the referred person, and to push against the 'that's not for us' dialogue that's so common in services these days.

There is a powerful dialogue in services around gatekeeping, eligibility for services. It's uncomfortable saying 'no' but knowing there is nothing else for the person to access either. I hear narratives of 'We don't work with ... . x ... y ... z' and there seems to be a shutting down of thinking. Systemic conceptualisations can help us to challenge when the dialogue is 'What is the primary need for this person?'. Deconstructing a narrative of someone 'not fitting' can reframe the process.

Service models

There are lots of narratives in services of 'throughput... episodes of care'. I feel I need to fight for the space and time to be curious.

There is an increasing focus on contact time in services, and a dilemma of how to capture systemic liaison and non-direct work. We try to demonstrate the complicatedness and multi-agency nature of the work by making internal referrals to mark the multiple episodes of care from different professionals involved.

What influences the decision making around referrals? Does the label 'learning disability' influence these decisions? What is the service response to a 'revolving door' referral? – what assumptions are made, what is the role of stigma, can reasonable adjustments be made? How do we contract and make transparent the different service offerings and fully engage those referred in this process rather than this just being service led?

*Service models tend to be set up using an either/or frame (e.g. services either for learning disability **or** mental health needs). This can create a dilemma around how to get the person/problem into a shared space. Although many services might have narratives around joint work and integration, sometimes working across service boundaries can feel maverick and leave us wondering, 'Is it OK to share this space?'*

Measuring change

Another current service dialogue is measuring change. Many linear measures will provide a numerical score, so we need to help the service capture systemic change meaningfully. Using systemic measures and setting goals that capture change in the system is important so we can evidence that our practice is achieving good outcomes.

There is lots of work around a referral. Referrals will trigger all the service-demanded tools that are expected to be completed as a priority (such as questions around risk, nature of accommodation, employment) which can impact on the ability to develop a connection, and be creative and thoughtful about pacing. Instead, curiosity around the referral opens up a wider meaning-making dialogue and can balance service demands with being 'led' by the client/referrer.

How good are we at articulating what we've achieved with a referral, and how do we demonstrate shifts and changes that are wider than the referred person alone when services are designed to see the client or their diagnosis as the problem?

Person-centred

Another dilemma is the narrative in services about being 'person-centred'. Practitioners may want to involve others but there may be a sense again of being either/or rather than both/and. So, for example, taking a position of 'The focus of my work is with my client', rather than 'I can work with my client and also be thoughtful about how to include others'. There's a need to acknowledge that even individual work will impact on others in the system around the person.

Although we think about the referral being the start of the process it does have a journey and as part of that an ending. What was the journey before the referral was made? What have been the demands on the way? As part of the assessment or triage of the referral we need to also consider where it's been, who it's talked to, the experience and relationships to help, to really put the referral into a context. An example might be of a referral for a client with depression. Although this might be the start of the journey with our service for this episode of care, we might want to explore whether they have used our service before and what was their experience of it. What led them to seek help now? Who did they have to talk to for the referral to be made? Did it take courage, motivation, pressure from others to perhaps talk to their GP? Did the referral come straight to the Learning Disability service, or has it been declined by other services first such as the Community Mental Health Team? What meaning did the referred person and others make of that? What led them to persevere rather than give up? Who else knows about the depression? How has it impacted upon them? Have they been part of the help-seeking process?

The system around the person

What is 'family'? Does this definition shift for some people with learning disability? Family might have become a long-stay institution, or the paid service around a person, but does the system, albeit family or organisation around the person, see themselves as part of the process of change? Will, for example, carers understand how they can join with the client in systemic therapy and contribute to developing new ways of relating together and reducing the impact of the problem?

Referral also creates another system that involves those responding to it. Where is the emotion in the system? What is the professional response? Dilemmas arise around boundaries but also sharing communication: 'I'm here to work with Joe not his dad', 'Are we allowed to work in this way...we're supposed to work with Joe and be person-centred but without including others in the wider system no change can occur'. Rather than creativity being stifled by bureaucracy we need to open space to nurture it between us.

Reflective practice for staff involved

The goal may be to get a systemic thread through the work. Concerns about assessing and managing any risks tend to influence our speed/style of response, but the manner in which we ask questions can be systemic whilst still being attentive to ensuring everyone is kept safe.

It is not uncommon in a CTLD meeting for professionals to say to one another about a client something like 'I ended up involved' or 'I should have withdrawn weeks ago'. In these situations systemic thinking and skills can be so helpful to help reflect on the purpose of their involvement. Does it relate to client need or something else? For example, by helping practitioners to think about what has drawn them to remain involved, the conversation might develop an understanding of anxiety in the system, or by widening the lens/focus of a formulation that has become stuck (e.g. by asking questions about the wider context or including the perspectives of others that previously might not have been included), new ways of understanding and moving forward can be opened up. A systemic reflection around the referral can clarify roles and dilemmas.

It comes back to the nature of the referral – who and what are we referring and to whom? We usually receive a referral for a person but in fact it is the system that needs support. We may allow Joe into the service, but not those around him (they need the Relate door, Child and Family door and so on). How can we make connections with other services and reflect upon the professional practices that may limit or contribute to change? How can we work together?

Concluding reflections

Drawing on the reflections of colleagues, the value of adopting a systemic focus right from the very outset can be clearly highlighted. The lives of individuals with learning disabilities are often strongly influenced by both family and professional networks, and the usefulness of considering a referral without reflecting on the individual's wider system therefore becomes questionable. The consideration of referrals from a systemic standpoint prompts an entirely different way of thinking. Part of the challenge of our work is maintaining a person-centred focus whilst considering the complexity of all those influencing parts and people in the system around the client, and thinking about the referral from multiple perspectives. Systemic approaches bring a contextual richness to the lives of those we work with, ultimately allowing us to view a referral through a relationally focused lens. As humans, our lives are embedded within context. Why then, should we consider a referral, merely a snapshot into an individual's life, in the absence of such context? By thinking systemically right from the initial referral stage we immediately challenge the common assumption that the 'problem' is located within the individual, and instead afford an opportunity to consider alternative ways of conceptualising the problem. The challenge for the practitioner is creating opportunities to explore complexity, balance multiple viewpoints and ensure that the voices of others do not quieten that of the individual with the intellectual disability.

Box 5.2 Reflective questions on referrals

- When was the last time your team considered how it receives referrals?

- In what way does your referral process shape what is considered, how and by whom?

- What has been stimulated in your thinking by the questions posed in this chapter?

- Whose voices, stories or positions are dominant in your referral process?

Acknowledgements

Thanks to Frances, Darren, Rose, Natasha, Jenny, Bethan and Bronwen for your reflections.

References

Allen, D., James, W., Evans, J., Hawkins, S. & Jenkins, R. (2005). Positive behavioural support: Definition, current status and future directions. *Tizard Learning Disability Review*, 10(2), 4–11.

Burnham, J.B. (1986). *Family Therapy*. London: Routledge.

Carter, E.A. & McGoldrick, M. (1980). *The Family Life Cycle: A Framework for Family Therapy*. London and New York: Gardner Press.

Gore, N.J., McGill, P., Toogood, S., Allen, D., Hughes, J.C., Baker, P. & Denne, L.D. (2013). Definition and scope for positive behavioural support. *International Journal of Positive Behavioural Support*, 3(2), 14–23.

Halliday, S. & Robbins, L. (2006). Lifespan family therapy services. In S. Baum & H. Lynggaard (eds), *Intellectual Disabilities: A Systemic Approach* (pp. 42–63). London: Karnac.

Hassiotis, A. (2014). Clinical and cost effectiveness of staff training in Positive Behaviour Support (PBS) for treating challenging behaviour in adults with intellectual disability: A cluster randomised controlled trial. *BMC Psychiatry*, 14(1), 14–24.

Hwang, Y.S. & Kearney, P. (2013). A systematic review of mindfulness intervention evaluation of the effectiveness of mindfulness in reducing symptoms of depression and anxiety. *Journal of Intellectual Disability Research*, 59, 93–104.

Idusohan-Moizer, H., Sawicka, A., Dendle, J. & Albany, M. (2015). Mindfulness-based cognitive therapy for adults with intellectual disabilities: An evaluation of the effectiveness of mindfulness in reducing symptoms of depression and anxiety. *Journal of Intellectual Disabilty Research*. Feb, 59(2), 93–104.

Kushlick, A., Trower, P. & Dagnan, D. (1997). Applying cognitive-behavioural techniques to the carers of people with learning disabilities who display challenging behaviour. In B.S. Kroese, D. Dagnan & K. Loumidis (eds), *Cognitive Behaviour Therapy for People with Learning Disabilities* (pp. 141–161). London: Routledge.

NICE (2015). *Challenging Behaviour and Learning Disabilities: Prevention and Interventions for People with Learning Disabilities Whose Behaviour Challenges*. NICE guideline NG11, published May 2015.

NICE (2016). *Mental Health Problems in People with Learning Disabilities: Prevention, Assessment and Management*. NICE guideline NG54, published September 2016.

NICE (2017). *Learning Disabilities: Identifying and Managing Mental Health Problems*. Quality standard QS142, published January 2017.

Payne, M. (2000). *Narrative Therapy: An Introduction for Counsellors*. London: Sage Publications.

Sturmey, P. (2004). Cognitive therapy with people with intellectual disabilities: A selective review and critique. *Clinical Psychology and Psychotherapy*, 11, 222–232.

White, M. (1989). *Selected Papers*. Adelaide: Dulwich Centre Publications.

White, M. (1995). *Re-authoring Lives: Interviews and Essays*. Adelaide: Dulwich Centre Publications.

Section II

Introduction

This section is about what helps us to decide what we do and how we do it.

Section 2 considers the impact of context on how we are able to make things happen. Each chapter explores the application of systemic ideas in a different context pertinent to people who have been labelled with a learning disability and those who support them.

Burnham referred to the level of *method*, which incorporates the ways in which activities happen and the 'organisational patterns or practice protocol used both to set forth and bring forth aspects of the approach' (Burnham, 1992, p. 5).

The ways in which services are organised and provided has a clear relationship with what can happen and how it can happen. The overarching function of your unit may be education, social care, health care, or all three if you are a parent or carer. Each of these different organisations (or families) will have its own *organisational context*; that is, a range of methods and structures that it can draw on for what it does and how things are done. In the case of organisations, this will also include policies, procedures and guidance that govern practice and professional activities. Families often have scripts and patterns that they follow too. The methods we use are also influenced by the *wider contexts* of society: politics and economics.

Similarly, services are designed and commissioned to work with specific groups of people about particular things, for example young people and children with learning disabilities and mental health needs; older people with dementia or adults with learning disabilities and unmet health needs. Of course, this means that there are often things that we are not able to do, or people who need support that may be outside the remit of our employing organisation or role. Thus as well as an organisational context we are also likely to have a *service delivery context* such as special school; multidisciplinary community team; residential service; assessment and treatment unit; or specialist behaviour service.

Context also incorporates the resources that are available to us, whether these are people, places or materials. It can be about something as simple as the spaces and buildings that we are able to book and how this may help or hinder the activities we would like to undertake; the number of staff who can commit to joining a conversation at the same time; home visits versus a clinic; or the number of hours we can spend working with someone.

Life stages and transitions are contexts in which we operate. In this way the journey to obtaining a diagnosis; moving from children's to adult services; exploring end-of-life care; or improving our practice and knowledge base are also contexts where specific considerations influence both what we do and how we do it.

Reference

Burnham, J. (1992). Approach – Method – Technique: Making distinctions and creating connections. *Human Systems: The Journal of Systemic Consultation & Management*, 3, 3–26.

6

Working in the Context of a Diagnosis: Systemic Practice and Autism Spectrum Conditions

Mark Haydon-Laurelut

Accessible summary

- This chapter will explore a systemic approach to making sense of diagnoses.

- The chapter will explore a particular diagnosis, that of autism spectrum condition.

- The chapter considers how we can think about diagnoses as descriptions.

This chapter focuses on a diagnosis of autism spectrum condition (ASC); however, we might have focused on other diagnoses including learning disability. The chapter does not provide a blueprint for practice but rather an exploration of how we might think systemically about and practice in relation to the context of diagnosis.

The diagnosis industry produces descriptions called 'diagnoses' and they become part of the social world. They become part of the terrain within which we make sense of ourselves and others. Peter Stratton notes that 'because the diagnosis industry has so far been constructed on the assumption of deficiency within an individual, it is antithetical to systemic thinking' (Stratton, 2009, p. 3). As practitioners we will, however, encounter diagnoses and be required to make decisions about how we make sense of and relate to them. As descriptions and practices, any diagnoses can be thought of and practised systemically.

Diagnoses are social constructions. They are historically and temporally specific. This is not to say they cannot provide us with vitally important information, for example about a person's physical health, but rather that they are also descriptions that are created by particular communities of knowers sanctioned to create such diagnostic knowledge, and that this knowledge changes over time and across cultures. In 1992 one could still be diagnosed with homosexuality, and if we look back to the nineteenth century we encounter drapetomania, a condition characterised by the desire to escape from slavery. Descriptions that come to be called diagnoses are concerned with difference. Diagnoses reflect their cultures of origin, and in the case of drapetomania a culture of racism. Diagnostic criteria for ASC have altered considerably over recent years, beginning with the third edition of the Diagnostic and Statistical Manual (DSM) of the American Psychiatric Association, gaining and subsequently losing associated spectrum disorders such as Pervasive Developmental Disorder – Not Otherwise Specified (PDD-NOS) (Denham-Boyce, 2014) and Asperger Syndrome (Hassall, 2016) along the way. ASC as a diagnosis has been interrogated in relation to its cultural, political and economic context (see, for example, Runswick-Cole et al., 2016). In widening our view of a diagnosis we may create new meanings and possibilities for action. For example, Timimi et al. (2011, p. 7) place Autism (sic) in the context of historical, economic and political change, producing a description of Autism (sic) as a 'metaphor for focusing on a disparate range of behaviours that suggest a lack of the type of social and emotional competencies thought to be necessary for the functioning of societies dominated by neoliberal economic and political foundations'. Thus we see how broadening or changing the contexts in which we understand a diagnosis offers new ways of making sense of it.

Writing about and working with diagnostic descriptions: Eating the menu?

Writing about working with a specific diagnosis presents dilemmas that need to be addressed and may help us think about our work. Writing about a diagnosis risks foregrounding the diagnostic story. Basing our work on a diagnosis risks losing the individual and privileging knowledge created outside of their relational network and their unique, unfolding 'life course' (Grant, 2010).

There is a rich systemic tradition we can draw upon when we encounter diagnostic stories. This work enables us to be alert to invitations to accept that a diagnosis can unproblematically connect us to reality. Diagnoses are a 'map, not the territory' (Korzybski, cited in Ivanovas, 2007). What is meant by this? Systemic pioneer Gregory Bateson explored the issue, as noted by Ivanovas:

> Bateson stressed again and again that our concepts are something different from what is happening and confusing the two would be like eating the written menu in a restaurant (with all the fine meals written on) instead of waiting for the real menu.
>
> (Ivanovas, 2007, p. 848)

Ivanovas again:

> A diagnosis is a description of a certain human condition, mostly in terms of patho-physiological alterations ... However as soon as physicians start to treat a disease they have eaten the menu.
>
> (Ivanonas, 2007, p. 848)

To 'eat the menu' is to relate to a particular description as if it were more than a description or a description that takes precedence over any other. It is to mistake the map for the territory. Systemic theory and practice celebrates the importance of multiple descriptions or stories as bringing forth alternative 'menus' or meanings and possibilities for ourselves and those who consult us. We may find that the issues in the person's life that brought them to us as well as the changes they seek may have few connections with a diagnostic description.

The ecology of diagnosis

Adults with learning disabilities who have a diagnosis of ASC may have experienced trauma, may reside in inappropriate accommodation, may have experienced loss, may have experienced involuntary dislocation as they have been sent to 'hospitals' away from family and community, may be struggling to create a life and a positive sense of identity for themselves as a young adult or be adjusting to advancing age. They may receive too little support (this may have been reduced during the current government's policy of cutting funds to disabled people), be served by a service system that is disjointed and confusing for families, staff and clients alike, and may have difficulties related more generally to learning disability, both cognitively (memory, planning, language comprehension and so on) and associated with social responses to impairment (or negatively valued difference): oppression, poverty and psycho-emotional and structural disablism (Reeve, Chapter 3 of this volume). There will be quieter stories of abilities, hopes and dreams, individual interests, likes and dislikes.

They will all live within a unique web of relationships, resources and individuals. A diagnosis always lives in an ecology such as this.

Diagnosis as a context

A diagnosis may constitute a frame or story through which a person and others in a person's life (family, work colleagues, professionals and so on) are viewing the life of the person. A person's relationships, difficulties and sometimes abilities may come to be viewed through the lens of a diagnosis. The difficulties experienced may have led to a referral to a health or social care professional. The diagnosis might offer a way of interpreting the actions of the person. The person's actions may be seen to reflect an inner diagnostic reality. In framing the life of the person in this manner we may hear linear talk that describes a person as acting in a certain way *because* they have an autism spectrum condition. Diagnoses may, arguably, offer some information and, as systemic practitioners, we can also be interested in how this diagnosis may have been organising understandings and stories about a person.

Referrals and diagnoses as possibilities

A referral is made by someone who considers there is a problem or difficulty that requires attention and so the stories of the referrer and the interactions between referrers and the referred person are also of interest. Turning these problem-focused descriptions on their head can assist us in responding creatively to referrals. Systemic psychotherapist Peter Lang understood that 'every problem is a frustrated dream'. For Lang, when we encounter problem descriptions we can choose to understand them as dreams that may not yet have been realised. We can choose to ask about the problem or about the dream. If we consider concerns that might be expressed in relation to diagnosis (e.g. about whether a new diagnosis is required, if the person is receiving the correct support for the diagnosis or questions about the extent to which a person might live an 'ordinary' life with a diagnosis), these are opportunities to explore the dreams and hopes; for example:

What would be your best hopes if a new diagnosis was received?

How would we know we were getting the support right for this person? What would we see in their lives? What would they be doing? Who would be with them?

Let us talk more about the life you have in mind for the person.

What might be the first step to bring this about?

This kind of focus acknowledges the hopeful intentions of the person and their supporters, does not directly challenge the importance of diagnosis for them and offers space to discuss 'the dream' in greater detail than the diagnostic conversation might permit.

Widening the view

What if we were to consider a diagnostic description as a story that provides a context for making sense? It may be a useful context for some in particular moments, and less so in others. Working systemically can draw attention to many other contexts to create rich understandings and stories. What kinds of contexts? These may be contexts influencing the difficulties that lead to a referral, such as changes taking place in the referring service; changes in family circumstances of the person; disruption and reduction of the person's or their family's finances; relationship breakdown; poor nutrition; a sensory issue; or poor quality housing, to name just a few. We may ask about the context of time. How were difficulties and hopes experienced and understood at earlier times and how are they being imagined into the future? These are linked with wider contexts of culture, economy and the political landscape. As we widen our view, zooming out (Bateson, 2017) to view a referral through the multiple contexts that make up and frame a life, we do not seek to remove or discredit the diagnostic context but rather it is joined by other contexts and re-contextualised as one meaning among many.

Being curious about diagnoses

A diagnosis (map) may be something different from what is happening in the world (territory) of the person we work with. However, diagnoses *are* happening. They are powerful maps, stories that influence and organise meanings. They may be present in the texts of referrals (Nunkoosing & Haydon-Laurelut, 2011), in the discussion in a meeting or in the professional notes and assessments that have taken place. A diagnosis risks punctuating (or even blaming) one person for the difficulties that a system of people may be experiencing. We can ask after Rikberg Smyly (2006), 'Who needs to change?' This is not to invite confrontation, but as Robbins (Chapter 5 of this volume) shows, it is rather to explore the ways in which the idea that help was required, that change was sought, came about.

Sometimes a diagnosis might feel like a kind of 'full stop' (Bateson, 1972, p. 39). It can be likened to a signpost saying 'Stop, look no further!'. A diagnosis is a description; there is always more to see and know, other contexts to explore. Life and our shared ideas about it change, evolve and develop. For Nora Bateson (2016, 2017) this appreciation of living complexity is an ethical issue: 'I would like to protect all living, growing, evolving processes from the violence of being freeze-framed. I stand by the dignity of living complexity.' (Bateson, 2016, p. 207) I have noticed ASC (and many other concepts) used as an explanatory principle. What is an explanatory principle? Gregory Bateson contrasted explanatory principles with hypotheses as follows: 'an hypothesis tries to explain some particular something but an explanatory principle – like gravity or instinct – really explains nothing. It's a sort of conventional agreement between scientists to stop trying to explain things at a certain point.' (Bateson, 1972, p. 39). Might we notice the places where we, a person, a family or a wider community and/or professional network have stopped trying to explain things? Have we settled on a single description? We can use our curiosity and ask about the description. We can explore multiple contexts (such as by mapping changing views over time and between persons, looking through the lens of various theories or the lens of exceptions, by employing new language and putting current terms aside, and so on), and in doing so support the co-creation of richer, multiple descriptions and possibilities.

Duelling realities

Sometimes there are 'duelling realities' (Anderson, 1997), where stories of family life, the nature of the problem and the shape of possible solutions are a matter of profound disagreement. As systemic practitioners we are less interested in who has the correct description of the world (whether a person has autism or not, who is to 'blame' for this or that difficulty and so on) and more focused on finding ways of being with people that will be useful for them. This can lead us to ask about what is important to people and what is wanted as we thicken stories of value and future. A diagnosis and the characteristics it might imply may or may not be particularly salient to this kind of conversation. In exercising our curiosity about the ecology of diagnoses we can notice how they might influence and organise. Do they draw us away from a consideration of other contexts? Might they in our busy working lives offer us a 'short circuit' (Bateson, 2017) to 'understanding'? We can enquire as to how they came about. Bianciardi and Bertrando (2009, p. 98) ask what a clinician, in concert with a person and members of their network, has engaged in that made the bestowing of a particular diagnosis possible:

> Within our logic, it makes no sense to wonder whether a diagnosis is right or wrong, but rather to wonder how that diagnosis emerged within that encounter: how the relationship between therapist and patient created such a context to favour the emergence of that specific diagnostic criterion, instead of other ones? Why did not the therapist see other data? And how did the patient present him- or herself to the therapist as a patient who could be framed within those diagnostic criteria?
>
> (Bianciardi & Bertrando, 2009, p. 98)

In place of considering whether a diagnosis is correct (using a logic of either/ or) we can explore and take response-ability for how it was that a professional and client system co-created a context in which the diagnostic practices took place.

Curiosity (Cecchin, 1987) invites us to become interested in the ways in which clients make sense of and tell stories about their worlds. We also invite them to become interested in their own stories, lived (the patterns of interaction they engage in) and told (the way they describe and make meaning). In asking curious questions we can invite people to enquire about the life of a diagnosis. As diagnoses may powerfully impact on the lives of those who receive them and on those who are significant to those diagnosed, an interrogation of diagnoses is warranted:

> [T]his raises questions regarding consent to diagnosis of disabled people with learning difficulties. What are the risks of diagnosis – to the individual, to their family, to the community and the wider culture? How as clinicians should we be assessing these risks? How is capacity to give or withhold consent to the diagnostic process negotiated with adults with more severe learning difficulties?
>
> (Haydon-Laurelut, 2016, p. 235)

However, we should be wary of disregarding diagnoses. We can be curious about the instrumental function of a diagnosis; for example, a diagnosis may play an important part in improving well-being by enabling the diagnosed person to obtain support from services. A fixed ideological position (for or against) diagnosis in a general sense leaves us with little flexibility when meeting with clients who do not share our views (or, indeed, meeting with those whose views we share – how can we then introduce a useful difference of perspective?).

But a systemic view of diagnosis calls for the exploration of more than one context. Life is a complex and ever-changing ecology. To think systemically is to honour this complexity and consider its many interdependencies (see Bateson, 2016). A diagnosis may, for example, both offer the possibility of access to resources (or not) and have consequences (preferred or not) for the identity of the person diagnosed, their social identity, family relationships and the stories and possibilities available to them throughout life. A diagnosis may be desired by one family member and not others. It may appear desirable now and also harbour unknown consequences. These may be very difficult and complex decisions and conversations for persons with learning disability, their families and supporters to navigate. This further highlights the importance of taking a curious position about the multi-contextual reverberations of diagnoses.

What might a diagnosis of ASC mean to the person and their family and network of relationships? Consider the following questions:

How might a diagnosis of ASC contextualise stories of the person's (and their family's) future, their support, their possibilities of relationships in adulthood and their work life?

How is a network's understanding of ASC influencing how they are making sense of a person's distress?

More specifically:

Is anxiety viewed as something that is endemic to ASC? Does this stop or encourage exploration of the best ways to support the person? How can anxiety be the start of an exploration about the person and their support?

Is curiosity about distress stymied by a story of 'autistic meltdown'? How might it be a useful concept to the person and their family? What other contexts can be added to enrich our descriptions of what is happening? (See Chapter 20, 'Diversity IS GRACE'.)

How are descriptions (in the example here, 'anxiety' or 'autistic meltdown') useful to the person and their supporters and when they are less so? We might ask about the contexts of anxiety such as when it occurs and when the word 'anxiety' was first used, and what other words might be used if we put the word to one side for a moment (questions I encountered through the workshops of the late Peter Lang); what encourages anxiety, what keeps it in check and when it is useful as a message that something needs to change (see Chapter 5 for more detail on these kinds of questions), and so on, can help a person and their network develop flexibility in the face of a difficulty. It is a reminder of the 'living, growing, evolving processes' (Bateson, 2016, p. 207) involved in the lives of those who consult with us.

Exploring knowledges

Knowledge as described by Nunkoosing (2000, 2012 and in Chapter 2 of this volume) is socially constructed and hence, as it changes across time and cultures, exists in multiplicities. What 'ASC knowledges' do those that consult us possess? That ASC is a pathology to be cured; a valued form of neuro-diversity; an administrative category to which one submits in order to receive support? Different family members may be living out subtly or dramatically different knowledges and these may differ also from professionals involved, who may believe they have authoritative scientific stories of ASC that take precedence over those of clients and their families (See Runswick-Cole et al., 2016) for a critique of the scientific basis of ASC and alternative conceptions). If differences remain unknown, unspoken, untellable or unheard (Rascon & Littlejohn, 2017), those working together following a referral may struggle to coordinate their meanings and actions. If this is the case, exploring relationships to diagnoses may support those who consult with us to notice and make sense of these potentially powerful descriptions of themselves and their family and network. An important aspect of this is learning to notice what kind of knowledge may be influencing us at particular moments and how this may be useful for particular clients.

Considerations

This chapter has offered an account of diagnoses as descriptions. These descriptions and related practices are part of the ecology of cultures, institutions, professions, relational networks, families and the inner conversations of personal identity. As such, diagnoses are, like all descriptions, the map not the territory (Korzybski, cited in Ivanovas, 2007). I have offered an approach to descriptions known as diagnoses that does not seek to refute or privilege them but rather to outline a multi-contextual understanding stance where one holds open a space of curiosity about their niche in individuals' lives. A contemporary systemic approach to this issue must include an acknowledgement of power and privilege, and diagnostic descriptions are privileged, powerful descriptions. This chapter has considered the importance of being mindful of this power as we support those who consult us to navigate diagnoses. The chapter will conclude with some suggested reflexive questions that may assist your thinking about relationships to diagnosis.

Box 6.1 Reflective questions on diagnosis (these questions can be thought about in relation to any diagnosis)

Questions about a person you are supporting

In what ways might a diagnosis of X speak to others about the person's identity?

What might this diagnosis obscure?

What is the life of the diagnosis in the person's life? In what ways might the diagnosis help us towards useful understandings of this person? In what ways might it lead us away from useful understandings the person?

What does this diagnosis appear to be telling the person about themselves? What (if anything) might be done about this?

How is the person, and those in their life, relating to the diagnosis? What is this creating? How can you find out about how they might wish to relate to it?

Self-reflexive questions exploring your relationship to diagnoses

What diagnosis stories are there in your family?

How have you related/might you relate to receiving a diagnosis or not receiving one?

Think of a diagnosis you are familiar with (one that you own or one that someone that you know does). What traits do you associate with that diagnosis? Now think of someone else who has those traits but no diagnosis. What might people in these two situations learn from each other?

Is gender a diagnosis assigned at birth?

If drapetomania reflected a culture of racism, what is reflected in the particular diagnosis you are encountering in your work?

References

Anderson, H. (1997). *Conversation, Language and Possibilities: A Postmodern Approach to Therapy*. New York: Basic Books.

Bateson, G. (1972). *Steps to an Ecology of Mind*. London: The University of Chicago Press.

Bateson, N. (2016). *Smaller Arcs of Larger Circles*. Axminster, UK: Triarchy Press.

Bateson, N. (2017). Warm Data. https://norabateson.wordpress.com/2017/05/28/warm-data (accessed 25 August 2018).

Bianciardi, M. & Bertrando, B. (2009). Ethical therapy: A proposal for the postmodern era. Human systems. *The Journal of Therapy Consultation and Training*, 20(2), 87–101.

Cecchin, G. (1987). Hypothesizing, circularity, and neutrality revisited: An invitation to curiosity. *Family Process*, 26, 405–413.

Denham-Boyce, L. (2014). Autism through the years. *PsyPAG Quarterly*, 93, 50–53.

Grant, G. (2010). Family care: Experiences and expectations. In G. Grant, P. Ramcharan & M. Flynn (eds), *Learning Disability: A Life Cycle Approach* (pp. 171–183). UK: Open University Press.

Hassall, R. (2016). Does everybody with an autism diagnosis have the same underlying condition? In K. Runswick-Cole, R. Mallett & S. Timimi (eds), *Re-Thinking Autism: Diagnosis, Identity and Equality* (pp. 49–66). London: Jessica Kingsley Publishers.

Haydon-Laurelut, M. (2016). Critical systemic therapy: Autism stories and disabled people with learning difficulties. In K. Runswick-Cole, R. Mallett & S. Timimi (eds), *Re-Thinking Autism: Diagnosis, Identity and Equality* (pp. 221–238). London: Jessica Kingsley Publishers.

Ivanovas, G. (2007). Still not paradigmatic. *Kybernetes*, 36(7–8), 847–851.

Nunkoosing, K. (2000). Constructing learning disability: Consequences for men and women with learning disabilities. *Journal of Learning Disabilities*, 4(1), 49–62.

Nunkoosing, K. (2012). The social construction of learning disability. In H.L. Atherton & D.J. Crickmore (eds), *Learning Disabilities: Towards Inclusion* (pp. 3–16). London: Churchill Livingstone.

Nunkoosing, K. & Haydon-Laurelut, M. (2011). Intellectual disabilities, challenging behaviour and referral texts: A critical discourse analysis. *Disability & Society*, 26(4), 405–417.

Rascon, N.A. & Littlejohn, S.W. (2017). *Coordinated Management of Meaning (CMM): A Research Manual*. Chagrin Falls, OH: Taos Institute.

Rikberg Smyly, S. (2006). Who needs to change? In S. Baum & H. Lynggaard (eds), *Intellectual Disabilities: A Systemic Approach* (pp. 42–63). London: Karnac.

Runswick-Cole, K., Mallett, R. & Timimi, S. (eds) (2016). *Re-Thinking Autism: Diagnosis, Identity and Equality*. London: Jessica Kingsley Publishers.

Stratton, P. (2009). Editorial. Human systems. *The Journal of Therapy Consultation and Training*, 20(2), 2–5.

Timimi, S., Gardner, N. & McCabe, B. (2011). *The Myth of Autism: Medicalising Men's and Boys' Social and Emotional Competence*. Basingstoke: Palgrave Macmillan.

7

Systemic Ideas in the Context of Working with Children, Young People and Families

Sarah Brown, Leanne Coleman, Katarina Luce and Jennifer McElwee

Accessible summary

In this chapter, we talk about:

- our experiences with children and young people with a label of learning disabilities

- how important children and young people and their families are in making change in their own lives

- how we can help people connect with each other and work together

- supporting children and young people with a label of learning disabilities and their families to be valued community members.

This chapter draws directly on the experiences and ideas of children, young people, parents and carers and practitioners, and views them as people who bring valuable expertise, and not as 'problems' defined by 'expert' systems of support, or 'patients' in need of 'help'. The chapter presents a strong argument for collaboration and mutual respect between children, young people, their families and practitioners, with each person viewed as bringing something of value to the relationship.

Hayley (1976) suggests that defining a problem in relation to an individual could be considered narrow and unpalatable, whereas defining problems as economic and cultural could lead the practitioner to become a revolutionary, leaving the client to wait in distress whilst the practitioner organises the revolution. We relate to this and see a fundamental tension present in our work with children and young people with a label of learning disabilities, their families and support systems. Working with children with a label of learning disability can be about more than promoting emotional well-being and reducing distress; when social justice is a value in our work, it can expose issues of power and create new possibilities for social systems to be supportive and resist oppression.

This chapter frames systemic ideas in the context of working with children, young people and families by presenting three case studies. Leanne (mum of two children, one of whom has the labels of learning disability and autism) talks about her experience of being a parent and what the labels have meant for her. Jeni (clinical psychologist) presents work with a group of young people with a label of learning disability. Katarina (mother of three young children, one of whom has complex needs) presents a community initiative, SENDawelcome (SEND is an acronym for special educational needs and disabilities).

Leanne's story

When our son, Charlie, was six months old, I had a gut feeling that something was different with his development compared to our eldest son. He didn't really cry; when I tried to interact with him I didn't get anything back, like he didn't know I was there. I didn't mention it to anyone, because who wants to be the first to say it? Then the day Charlie's health visitor told me that he might have autism, I didn't know anything about it; I asked her if it was life-threatening. I really didn't know what would follow. I remember her saying, 'It's going to be OK, I'm here to support you.' I remember her saying that I wouldn't be able to help Charlie until I could help myself; until I could accept Charlie for who he was. She told me not to put pressure on myself and allow myself to experience cycles of different emotions.

I decided that if this was how our life was going to be I wanted to find ways to help Charlie be happy and make things easier for him. I started to read books and ask questions. Having Charlie made me think about the way that I communicate. I don't think I was patient before. I had to slow my pace down, and not rush around. I had to change my language so that Charlie understood me. I remember feeling like this was my priority, that nothing else mattered. I felt like my employment was just something to pay the bills and my job was to learn about autism. At the beginning, I became a bit unwell with it. I didn't want to let him down. I didn't want him to feel like he was alone.

I also began to feel guilt towards Dylan, our eldest son. Was he getting what he needed from me in the way Charlie was? It seemed like there wasn't enough of me to go around. I wondered whether he felt the same as me when I was growing up and caring for my mother. In the beginning, I tried to protect him and didn't really tell him about Charlie's autism. Dylan asked me if Charlie was dying because we had all these appointments at the hospital. We realised that he would make sense of what was going on if we were honest. Now, I give Dylan opportunities to talk about his feelings. He doesn't have to feel alone, any emotion that he experiences is warranted and important. I want him to be able to express everything and know we'll accept it.

At the beginning of our life with Charlie there were times when we struggled with feeling isolated and separate from our family and community. When I dropped Charlie in nursery the 'mainstream' class turned right and the children with 'communication issues' went to the left. I felt very different to the other parents, and I felt that others were looking at me with sorrow. Some parents would make quite a big fuss of Charlie and others wouldn't want to look at all. The staff were brilliant, really nurturing.

On one occasion, I went to the GP with Charlie and he was finding it difficult in the waiting room. He didn't have any language so he was screeching and couldn't sit still. A lady said to me: 'He's lovely, how old is he? He's just like our grandson.' The man with her said, 'He's nothing like our grandson – she can't even control him.' I felt that Charlie didn't deserve that and neither did we. After this we started to stay at home more. I was wary of other people's reactions.

Yet I didn't want us to be isolated; I wanted to educate people. We started going back out into the community with my friend and her children, until I felt more confident. Then I met up with other parents of children with learning disabilities. Eventually I decided to do some fundraising for a local charity for disabled children. It felt like this was my way of introducing Charlie's autism into my community in a positive and fun way. I did a sponsored zip wire event with five of my friends and my eldest son. I contacted the local paper myself. It was my way of saying, 'Yes he is different and that's OK.' I felt more comfortable after that, and it helped to shape other people's reactions to us.

Sometimes as a parent I can't help but feel so sad, and my heart hurts so much, because I see children the same age as my son who I've known for years, whose lives are taking a very different path to Charlie's life. Then I stop and look back at my amazing boy, my son, and see his huge achievements! I see how far he has come, all he has been through. The little boy who couldn't speak, who struggled in so many areas of his life, to the boy who makes me smile today, who is finding his confidence and finding his feet in this challenging world, and in some ways or another is allowing us to hear his voice. Most importantly, I see a young man who is finding happiness and that hurt in my heart is turned into joy, because as a mother that's all I want for my children, because life isn't a competition is it? Life is what you make of it, regardless of whether you may need support or not, and nothing should stop you achieving your dreams, whatever they may be.

Some thoughts from Sarah and Jeni

Miller (1997) highlights two different kinds of 'searching' by parents and carers of children and young people with a label of learning disabilities. The first is *searching for information:* for assessment, sometimes diagnosis, and for intervention and support. Often, as for Leanne's family, a diagnosis is given within a medical framework and what can be appealing about this is the sense of certainty, of having some answers and being able to help. This can sometimes be experienced as a (usually temporary) relief, yet can also be a source of distress. Simon (2016) comments that the diagnostic process can position the family as a victim of unfortunate circumstances and give them advice to help 'cope' with their child (who has the problem within them); she says that what the professional system fails to see is the *family system* struggling to cope with communication challenges, and that it is 'resourceful, creative and open to collaborative approaches'. As Simon comments, the struggles that parents want help with are almost always relational. We see this in how Leanne framed her struggles with her son and the questions she really wanted help with: how do I build a relationship between Charlie and his community? How do I communicate with Charlie? How do I make sure I have time for both my children?

The second kind of searching that Miller (1997) describes parents as doing is *inner searching*: for the meaning of developmental differences for the child, for them as parents and them as a family. Meaning is influenced by context, including the family's sociocultural context and religious beliefs, their views of disability and their own experience of disability. Often, parents welcome a chance to think about the questions they are asking themselves but may fear speaking aloud – will my child have an 'ordinary' life? What kind of parent do I need to be? What does this mean for our relationships? Why has this happened to my child?

What Leanne describes are her own creative and thoughtful *relational solutions* to the challenges her family as a system faced. What we mean by this is that instead of seeing Charlie as the 'problem' in need of individualised treatment, her focus was on building positive communication between family members and the community, and drawing on positive aspects of existing relationships (particularly her friendships) to support her. Leanne found a way to put herself in her son's shoes and change her communication so they could understand each other, then she shared this with the rest of the family. She considered how her eldest son's position and role within the family had shifted and connected this to her own story of being in a caring position as a child. She found a way to talk to her eldest son, and be open to accepting all his feelings. She found a way to manage rejection and hostility in the community by building her confidence with the help of a friend, and eventually by being brave enough to speak to the whole community via a newspaper article and fundraising.

Leanne talks about the structural barriers (in terms of turning left to go to a separate part of the nursery) and social barriers (being publicly shamed for her son's distress) that her family have faced. She internalises the oppression and stays away from the community, until she finds her own strategies to manage the emotional reactions of others and potential social rejection. Runswick-Cole (2013) talks about this kind of strategy as 'emotional labour', defined as when 'a person is hiding or changing his or her feelings to show a more acceptable emotional front to those around them'. She talks about the emotional labour for disabled children and their parents as they induce or suppress feelings and absorb others' emotions to conform to normative social scripts. She suggests that at times parents may change their behaviour in response to the perceived emotional labour that could occur otherwise. Leanne took a brave step in managing the reactions of others very publicly, through raising money for a charity and letting people know about her son's needs. In this sense, she was the voice not just for her and her son, but also for other families who live with a label of learning disability and autism.

Box 7.1 Reflective questions on families

- How can you describe child or family 'problems' in relational terms in order to support families to find relational solutions?

- In what contexts can you highlight the possible impact of emotional labour in order to create new conversations?

- How can you highlight structural and social barriers faced by families in order to shift the focus from a within-child problem to a system and social problem?

Jeni's story

Members of our team (a community mental health team for children with learning disabilities) visit a group of young people with a label of moderate to severe learning disabilities who all attend the same specialist educational setting. We meet once a month with the aim of hearing and responding to the young people's views about our service. Our employer, the National Health Service (NHS), calls this 'participation' (NHS England, 2017). The young people have a range of communication needs and over time we have learnt that we need to conceptualise our sessions in two separate parts if we want to have a meaningful

*conversation. Firstly, we think about promoting and developing the young peo-
ple's 'voice' (where 'voice' means what the young people think about the world
and is not synonymous with verbal communication). Secondly, we have 'conversations' about what the young people think about the world in general and health
services in particular (where 'conversations' often means presenting a situation
and observing a response, rather than a series of words only).*

Voice

*Sessions have a predictable structure, comprising a start section (with intro-
ductory music, introduction of the young people's 'leader' of the session and
a reminder of rules), a 'voice' section and a 'conversation' section, followed by
summary and ending music. The predictable structure supports young people
to know what is happening next and we have seen all the young people in the
group step up confidently to take the 'leader' role, even those who generally
keep quiet. Our rules are 'You say and show,' and 'We listen'. We all take part
in activities to promote the idea that everybody's views are important. In the
'voice' section the leader presents the group with a series of objects that stimu-
lates each of the five senses (e.g., bubbles for vision and tinned fish for smell).
We ask people to point to a green card with a tick for 'like' and a red card
with a cross for 'don't like'. We respond positively to both responses as we are
hoping to promote a sense of ownership over each person's point of view. Over
time we have seen some people move from hesitancy to clear expression of their
likes and dislikes. One young woman pointed to 'like' for every stimulus over a
number of sessions and it was a moment of celebration when she first expressed
her dislike.*

Conversation

*We use our 'conversation' section to continue to ask the group questions, listen
to their response, and show them we have listened by responding ourselves.
We started the group by looking through some pictures to decide what the group
was going to be called and then created a large group logo in the middle of a
table, which was reduced in size and printed on T-shirts for everybody to wear
during subsequent groups. Then we asked the group to carry cameras around
the school and take photos of things they liked and didn't like and, if possible, to
record why. The group stuck the pictures on pieces of paper signalling 'like' and
'don't like' and fed back to the school, which made changes. Recently we went
to a health centre to take photos and interview staff using questions prepared in
advance by the young people and ideas will be fed back to the health centre in the
coming months.*

Some thoughts from Sarah and Jeni

When we talk about including the 'voice' of all children and young people it can be tempting to engage only with those who can express themselves verbally with ease. Goodley (2001) discusses a view within critical disabilities research that appears to reflect a distinction between the labels of 'mild' and 'severe' learning disabilities, such that 'mild learning disabilities' is seen as socially constructed, whereas those labelled as having 'severe learning disabilities' are excluded and thought of as having an impairment that is static and biologically based. Simmons and Watson (2014, 2015) highlight and challenge this assumption in their work with a young person labelled with 'profound and multiple learning disabilities' (PMLD). They suggest that people so labelled are primarily described in terms of developmental deficits, such as being pre-verbal, pre-volitional and pre-symbolic (the person does not intentionally communicate meaning to others). Simmons and Watson (2015) contrast these descriptions with definitions of 'personhood' that refer to being 'richly self-aware', 'linguistically competent' and 'highly social' and suggest that viewed within this frame, people labelled with PMLD are not identified as being people. We have noticed this viewpoint when working with young people labelled with 'profound and multiple learning disabilities', where it is not uncommon for systems of support to regularly exclude a young person from decisions about every aspect of their daily life due to a belief that the young person would be unable to contribute. Simmons and Watson (2015) suggest that a way of introducing a discourse about the social nature of the label of 'PMLD' would be to widen (refocus?) the lens on what it means to be a person. Their ideas influence the way we work, and help us to challenge some of the disabling discourses that we and others may bring into the room.

> **Box 7.2 Reflective questions on promoting children's voices**
>
> In your work:
>
> Who do you invite to contribute and how do you invite them to contribute?
>
> How do you ensure that children and young people know they have a voice and that this voice is heard (particularly when they communicate without using language)?
>
> ▶

◀

Can you think of a time when you wanted to support a young person to express their views and it didn't go well?

What could you have done to support them to begin to understand what it is to have a voice and to begin to make choices?

Katarina's story

My son Gabe is rarely seen in our local community as he takes the bus to a specialist educational setting. Some local people don't know that I have a third child and generally people don't greet him if we go out. I became worried that a lifetime of people not saying 'hello' would teach my son to expect no 'Welcome'. I met with other parents of children with additional needs who live in our local community and we co-founded 'SENDawelcome', which is an initiative working towards authentic inclusion. We believe inclusion will happen when our children make meaningful connections with their community and are valued for their contributions within it. We want to activate a shift that ensures the community recognises and takes responsibility for including people with additional needs.

Although services are integral to supporting Gabe's needs, they are naturally fragile (due to budget constraints or staff simply leaving) and cannot be a substitute for Gabe developing long-lasting friendships. Staff in paid roles can create a barrier between Gabe and his community, as people see him as somehow 'sorted' and are therefore less inclined to view themselves as having a role to play in Gabe's life. Service involvement further labels Gabe as needing 'specialist' support that cannot be fulfilled by others. Gabe is in danger of missing out on what everyone needs – meaningful connections with those around him.

Visibility step by step

We aim to increase visibility through accessing shared community space. SENDawelcome is tackling this in a number of ways including meeting monthly in a local café with other families of children with additional needs. Crucially we have been working in a 'brokering' role between local facilitators of groups and activities and with families of children with additional needs. With providers we have established several 'accessible' sessions for families with a view to moving these children into the mainstream groups further down the line. This has been de-mystifying for both staff and for families who have deep-rooted, complex concerns about their children being involved in mainstream activities. There is always a danger that we become just another service provider that meets the needs of these children but perpetuates their invisibility by doing siloed activities separate from the rest of the community. We are also aware, though, that cultural change takes time, so we think about what we do as a series of steps towards our aim.

Education

Schools are at the centre of every local community. Specialist settings are currently seen as centres of excellence for promoting development in children with additional needs, but this system keeps children who are different from the norm separate. We think all children should have the opportunity to play and learn together, whilst still being aware that children need different types of support. Perhaps mainstream schools could become centres of excellence in inclusion? We would like schools to be recognised and rewarded for reflecting and representing those who make up a community. SENDawelcome is working towards providing training and learning experiences to children and staff in mainstream schools through drama workshops and discussion forums. This training will promote thinking around difference and how to familiarise the unfamiliar.

Celebration

All children are different but society is set up to view children with additional needs as extremely different. SENDawelcome is looking to celebrate achievements not relevant to social norms or milestones. We want to highlight the similarities between all children and celebrate the differences shown by children with additional needs, by inviting those differences into an acceptable and 'normal' arena.

Some thoughts from Sarah and Jeni

Haydon-Laurelut and Nunkoosing (2010) propose that in the present day 'people [with a label of learning disability] may live in the community, but they are rarely part of the community' (p. 74). In 2012, the government published *Transforming Care: A National Response to Winterbourne View Hospital* (Department of Health, 2012). This review was undertaken after an undercover investigation by BBC's *Panorama* programme revealed criminal abuse by staff at Winterbourne View Hospital of people with learning disabilities in their care. Events at Winterbourne View might suggest that the lives of people described as having learning disabilities have not changed dramatically since the time of institutions. Our experience would suggest that the situation is more complex than that; nevertheless, a consistent theme throughout the history of people described as having learning disabilities has been one of separation and segregation from society, either geographically, within institutions, and/or through disabling cultures, attitudes and sometimes abusive behaviours within society.

Rapley (2004) suggests that methods of assessment used by services socially construct both competence and incompetence. What and who others (and ourselves) are depends on our relationship with them and what we choose to make of the relationship. Haydon-Laurelut (2009) invites a service system to share 'response-ability' (when the expertise and resources within a service system are drawn upon) in the creation of and solution to problems. This fits with the values behind frameworks of support promoted by services such as Network Training (Jenkins & Parry, 2006) and Circles of Support (Burke & Ball, 2015). SENDawelcome wants to build upon this idea of service 'response-ability' by asking wider communities to accept children and young people with additional needs as valued and contributing members. Thus a young person can be someone who benefits from support *and* is a contributor. Systemic practitioners could reflect on and look beyond cultural discourses that encourage families to ask for support to think with families about how they could invite communities to see their child as a valued community member.

Box 7.3 Reflective questions on working in communities

- How do you motivate communities to take responsibility for those who live within them?

- How could you think with children and young people with additional needs and their families about social capital and contributing meaningfully to their community?

- What could you do to celebrate the lives of the children and young people you work with?

Conclusion: Systemic practice with young people with a label of learning disabilities

These are some ways in which we put systemic ideas into practice:

> Seeing relationships as fundamental to understanding the lives of the young people we work with.

> Thinking about how we position ourselves and others so that all 'voices' can be heard.

> Starting from a position of joining children and young people in their world and being curious about what this might look like.

> Being irreverent and thinking creatively about how to connect without using language as the main form of communication.

> Honouring parents as experts, whose lives are also being scrutinised by professional systems, and who we may be expecting to put on a 'brave face'.

> Situating systems of support within their cultural context and highlighting dominant narratives and enabling and disabling discourses.

> Promoting children and young people with a label of learning disabilities as valued community members.

> Creating new community narratives of celebration.

References

Burke, C. & Ball, K. (2015). *A Guide to Circles of Support*. London: Foundation for People with Learning Disabilities.

Department of Health (2012) *Transforming Care: A National Response to Winterbourne View Hospital*. London: Department of Health.

Goodley, D. (2001). 'Learning difficulties', the social model of disability and impairment: Challenging epistemologies. *Disability and Society*, 16(2), 207–231.

Haydon-Laurelut, M. (2009). Systemic therapy and the social relational model of disability: Enabling practices with people with intellectual disability. *Clinical Psychology and People with Learning Disability*, 7(3), 6–13.

Haydon-Laurelut, M. & Nunkoosing, K. (2010). 'I want to be listened to': Systemic psychotherapy with a man with intellectual disabilities and his paid supporters. *Journal of Family Therapy*, 32(1), 73–86.

Hayley, J. (1976). *Problem Solving Therapy*. London: Harper Collins.

Jenkins, R. & Parry, R. (2006). Working with the support network: Applying systemic practice in learning disabilities services. *British Journal of Learning Disabilities, 34,* 77–81.

Miller, N. (1997). *Nobody's Perfect: Living and Growing with Children Who Have Special Needs.* Maryland: Paul H. Brookes Publishing Co.

NHS England (2017). Patient and public participation policy. www.england.nhs.uk/publication/patient-and-public-participation-policy (accessed 8 January 2019).

Rapley, M. (2004). *The Social Construction of Intellectual Disability.* Cambridge: University Press.

Runswick-Cole, K. (2013). Wearing it all with a smile: Emotional labour in the lives of mothers and disabled children. In T. Curran & K. Runswick-Cole (eds), *Disabled Children's Childhood Studies: Critical Approaches in a Global Context* (pp. 105–118). Basingstoke and New York: Palgrave Macmillan.

Simmons, B. & Watson, D. (2014). *The PMLD Ambiguity.* London: Karnac Books.

Simmons, B. & Watson, D. (2015). Challenging the developmental reductionism of 'profound and multiple learning disabilities' through academic innovation. *PMLD Link, 263,* 25–27.

Simon, G. (2016). Thinking systems: 'Mind' as relational activity. In K. Runswick-Cole, R. Mallett & S. Timimi (eds), *Re-Thinking Autism: Diagnosis, Identity and Equality.* London and Philadelphia, PA: Jessica Kingsley Publishers, 269–287.

8

Evolving Educational (Psychology) Perspectives on Systemic Working

Julia Young, Ian Smillie and Amy Hamilton

Accessible summary

- We highlight the value of systemic thinking and working in education: *why do we want to work this way?*

- We consider the point of view of three different professionals (all educational psychologists) each in different roles: *how are we trying to do this?*

- We convey some of the challenges of working systemically within education and educational contexts: *what makes it difficult?*

- We show that despite the barriers and challenges, systemic thinking and working helps educational professionals have a more relational approach, which fits better than working in perceived 'traditional' (more linear) ways: *who benefits from this approach?*

Educational psychology is a relatively young profession that has been evolving for the past century. Broadly speaking, it is concerned with the application of psychology in education for the benefit of children and young people. Educational psychologists (EPs) are increasingly from a range of professional backgrounds and may work in different ways and in different contexts. In terms of the authors of this chapter, Julia works for a local authority where she works closely with school staff, Ian works in an early intervention service with families who have young children, and Amy works in a local authority with schools and has a particular interest in special schools. Ian and Amy are also professional tutors on an educational psychology doctoral training course.

The three of us strive to work systemically within our individual professional contexts, each holding our own construct of what it means to be systemic in our practice.

This chapter has developed through a process of dialogue between ourselves where we have had to acknowledge elements of our own discomfort and uncertainty regarding our position on systemic practice in education, and educational psychology in particular. For instance, how is it that we know best? And what if in the process of writing this chapter others perceive that we do? Therefore, the creation of this chapter has come from a place of discomfort – it was not easy. But to some degree this reflects the discomfort and difficulty of applying systemic ideas within an educational context. It's not easy.

Education is complex and messy. An EP is never just working with the 'education system', whatever that may be. There is not one simple or perceivable education system; it exists within a wider context of schools, communities, families, political agendas, local authorities, the medical world and so on. Within schools themselves, multiple systems exist that are both hard (e.g. targets and inspections) and soft (e.g. culture, relationships, emotional climate, family engagement, inclusion, community issues), and the 'problem' (which results in the involvement of an EP) never sits neatly within its own system. Any professional seeking to enable change in an educational context has to position themselves in a way that allows them to consider and explore all these systems.

Our perception of 'traditional' models of EP practice are that they are frequently linear in nature, akin to a medical or 'expert' approach. One obvious example is the use of psychometric testing and scores to enable access to specific resources; another is the 'expert' recommendations of EPs in their reports. Current models of EP practice – those used more recently in initial EP training – challenge traditional practice, for example of assessment to meet resource criteria and a within-child focus; some are social constructionist in their approach and include systemic thinking (e.g. the constructionist model of informed, reasoned action – COMOIRA – Gameson et al., 2003). This signifies the continually evolving nature of EP practice. However, it is clear that there is still much confusion among EPs about systemic thinking and working with systems (Fox, 2009). EPs are now qualified at doctorate level and on courses where systemic ideas are assumed, creating dilemmas such as having to both accept and deny an 'expert' position.

In the current climate of austerity, constraint and accountability, how do we facilitate systemic working when a linear approach appears less risky and onerous to others and therefore more favourable? Paradoxically, systemic EP work could offer better value for money in terms of avoiding lengthy assessments and subsequent reports that many professionals have little time to read, digest and utilise. In this sense there is a need to build trust with stakeholders, so that they understand and buy into the benefits of systemic work.

This chapter is concerned with working systemically in an educational context; fundamentally the authors come from a position that systemic practice can be beneficial to all stakeholders. Systemic thinking encourages inclusivity and collaboration, enables voices, especially perhaps of the more vulnerable, to be heard. The role of EPs is to promote change for the benefit of the more vulnerable in education (and therefore for all). Further, in rejecting the dominance of an expert model, our approach to this chapter is based upon sharing the authors' personal and professional perspectives, all three of which contain similar and overlapping themes regarding systemic working in education. We make no claim to offer answers but instead hope to inspire thought.

First, Julia considers her own understanding of systemic consultation as an EP and her struggle in working towards this. Then Ian spends some time reflecting on an element of his own attempts at systemic practice, specifically in relation to his work with a secondary school in challenging circumstances. Finally, Amy considers some of the complexities of working within a special school, the need for systemic practice in this context and the subsequent development of the Family Space project.

Systemic consultation (Julia Young)

My interest in systemic practice arises from a level of dissatisfaction and discomfort I experience in seeking to apply psychology within a system increasingly driven by measurement and targets. Systemic practice frees me to be a more collaborative professional working in an educational context.

Consultation is a large part of my work. Within our profession there is some confusion around the understanding and application of the terms 'consultation' (Fox, 2009; Nolan & Moreland, 2014), working at a 'systems level' and working 'systemically'. Systems level work in education contexts is that which goes beyond the individual child and aims to make change at a 'higher' level of the system, for example whole school training or work with a group of children. Systemic working might focus at any level; its difference is an awareness of the relations within the system around the child and between the child and those systems. Most educational psychology services (EPS) describe themselves as carrying out a 'consultation' model of service to schools. Such consultations are expected to promote or be a part of an intervention to help 'solve' a definable problem, within overarching, sometimes overt, targets, for example percentages of children or young people achieving a particular score/level in literacy and numeracy within a school or within the local authority as a whole. However, day-to-day practice of consultation varies between practitioners. For some EPs, consultation involves meeting and talking, often separately, with staff members and parents, then devising actions or 'recommendations' following those conversations and taking into account the 'referral' information. In this consultation work, hypothesising (i.e. generating ideas about what may be contributing to the way the problem arises and is understood) and problem solving can feel part of a linear and piecemeal process. We are invited to be experts coming to 'fix' a problem; sometimes that linearity feel may be unavoidable, as Ian clearly points out below. It may also be that the more relational (considering what happens between people and systems) content created by those conversations offers a more systemic approach, and that offers something new and useful within the linear process.

Systemic thinking includes trying to maintain curiosity. This means tolerating feelings of uncertainty (Mason, 1993) (e.g. I don't have the 'answer' and we may find one/several or none) and enabling others to do the same, as outlined in Amy and her colleagues' Family Space project below. This is a challenge. How do we deal with 'referral' (a linear term) information, thoughtfully written by teachers pushed for time? Part of the aim of requesting this information is to encourage others to hypothesise and to promote readiness for change. However, outside of a process of systemic consultation, this continues to appear as the referral (handing on) of a problem to an expert. Teachers (and perhaps parents) anticipating advice and unused to a systemic approach may sometimes feel they have not been provided with the concrete 'answer' they expected.

EPs often discuss working at a 'systems level' or carrying out 'systemic' work and use the phrases interchangeably. However, for me, systemic work is very different to 'working at a systems level' (though systemic work necessarily encompasses systems level working). Working at a systems level is about promoting change within a bigger system; professionals in an educational context may consider this appropriate when a wider need is perceived or when some part of that bigger system (a whole class, school, cluster of schools etc.) is seeking change. Often this involves structured work such as training or direct involvement with groups: for example, carrying out an approach such as Circle of Friends (a whole class approach to promoting social and emotional skills and improving relationships, Newton et al., 1996); or training teaching assistants to become ELSAs (emotional literacy support assistants). Systems work is often a very positive part of working as an EP and can create lasting and effective change, but it is not, in my view, the same as working systemically.

Systemic practice as an EP, I believe, involves differences in both the content and process of what I do on a daily basis. Realistically, this is an aspiration, something I am continually working towards and frequently distracted from (Amy and Ian both highlight their own similar struggles below). I interpret becoming increasingly systemic in my approach as valuing and highlighting relationships (Draeby, 1995), connections and differences. It is 'a curious consideration of multiple perspectives ... [involving] inclusion of context in exploring client problems, and ... [inviting] clients into an observer position on their own dilemmas' (Jones, 2003, p. 13). Utilising, for example, personal construct psychology (Moran, 2014), narrative (Freeman et al., 1997) and solution-focused (Rhodes & Ajmal, 1995) approaches in consultation meetings, as well as with children and young people, are some of the ways I feel able to use more of the (relational) psychology I value.

Hypothesising is an overt part of EP work which has the potential to involve many concepts of systemic consultation (e.g. context, positioning, feedback and circularity, observer position). In my own systemic consultation involving individual children, I will often observe and talk with a child or young person in class, then meet with all those (adults) involved with the 'problem'. The meeting is an opportunity for us all to share what we know about the child and the 'problem' and to come up with ideas to 'improve' the situation. During our discussions, I offer working hypotheses and ask parents and professionals for theirs and I ascertain their views of what they hear. I tend to seek children's views (as is consistent with law, guidance and policy, e.g. United Nations, 1989) and hypotheses, separately and through the adults in the meeting. Children and young people (YP) participating routinely in these daily consultation meetings would be a systemic ideal. Stakeholders sharing hypotheses is what I see as discovering relations: different perspectives, and how they might interact; how the relations(hip) between one person's ideas about what might be going on might affect another's. By promoting curiosity and having present as many of those involved with the problem as possible, each hears another perspective. It also offers opportunities to create reflections (Haselbo & Neilson, 2000) facilitated through maintaining neutrality (e.g. not accepting any particular hypothesis) and curiosity about the feedback and enabling everyone to be in an observer position. This is about dialogue; enabling listening and speaking for all those in the system; enabling the connections and differences to positively impact on the system. Evaluation of such approaches is achieved through a system of feedback and reflection within follow-up consultations, exploring questions such as: what has changed? What have you noticed that may be different? How come? In this way, our construction of what evaluation is shifts from a focus on what the professional may have done to help to actively considering the change that has occurred and what those most concerned may have done differently as a result of our work and thinking together.

Those who fully engage with EPs and other professionals in an education context who practise systemically will hopefully feel heard, understood and be a co-producer of the shared outcomes.

A spotlight on systemic practice in secondary schools (Ian Smillie)

Julia has already suggested some potential usefulness of a systemic consultation approach to professional practice in educational contexts. The relational element of such a way of working, it seems to me, can raise particular challenges for professionals within a secondary school context. This has certainly been my experience. I am motivated by Jones' (2003) description of the value of gaining multiple perspectives, of understanding the context through dialogue within those contexts, and inviting those we work with to take 'an observer perspective on their own dilemmas' (p. 13). Secondary schools can be extremely complex organisations, arguably more so than a family (Winslade & Monk, 2007); however, like families, schools are directly influenced by a range of other systems, and it is perhaps for this reason that systemic work in this context can be particularly challenging, yet ultimately worthwhile.

As a newly qualified educational psychologist, I began work with a secondary school within what was described by the head teacher as a 'deprived area'. The senior school staff with whom I was expected to most closely liaise described an expectation that I would come in to school and 'look at' a number of pupils who gave them reasons for concern. There was already an established process in place whereby the EP would be greeted by the additional learning needs coordinator (ALNCo) who would have already made arrangements for a discussion with a key staff member (in essence a verbal report and rarely a dialogue), a classroom observation and a meeting with the pupil. In my mind, this represented the traditional model of (often linear) EP working I felt so keen to move away from. This feeling was primarily based upon my interest in a *consultation* approach to educational psychology practice (Wagner, 2008), which advocates an *interactionist, constructionist* and *systemic* approach to applied psychological practice that reflects the complexity of educational contexts (what Wagner, 2008, refers to as 'inter-relating systems of schools, families, local-authority systems, professional systems, agencies, and so on' (p. 139)). I also had to respect that this is what was anticipated after the school's experience of previous people in this role. It was expected that a report would be written by the EP; very often this was considered the 'product' of the work, but a product that satisfied the needs of a system that reinforced a requirement, it seemed, to sort and classify pupils according to their need and to distribute funds and methods of 'support' accordingly. I became aware of my expected place in this process, and how this did not align with my own constructions of what it means to be a psychologist, a role, in my view, which was about helping people who are concerned to move towards some kind of real change, most usually, working with school staff, pupils and families to promote the understanding of pupil needs and the inclusion of pupils within mainstream learning environments. It concerned me that the school's historical approach seemed to qualify the pupil as a separate object of study from the systems that they occupied.

As my relationship with the school developed, colleagues would describe what they perceived as a significant problem within their school, that of poor and disruptive behaviour among the pupils, locating this confidently as the responsibility of the family or *the way they are brought up*. I found this interesting, because whilst there was a defined *response* of 'sending away' either internally (to another room) or externally (exclusion), the defined *solution* placed the concept of behaviour as arising from within the misbehaving individual rather than as something arising in a relational way. Consequently, my own attempts at trying to define and 'sell' a process of consultation, as Julia describes, felt ineffective as it was viewed that there was nothing in addition that the school could do, and instead the school began to invite the family in to meet with me as an additional part of the process – a kind of progress of sorts. What seemed clear, though, was that the young people I was asked to see tended to be 'repeat offenders', or those on the verge of permanent exclusion. I was struck by the pressure that this placed upon the process and upon my practice, and the hopelessness that this initiated in all concerned.

I wondered if the school had grown accustomed to a situation (a kind of 'homeostasis'), where Watzlawick et al.'s (1974) notion of 'Zero Sum Change' appeared to be relevant. The work of the educational psychologist and the school involved a process of 'ticking boxes' and this could be regarded as symptomatic of an organisation that was doing its best to cope. Attempts were made to deal with the situation based upon presumed causes, usually the pupil's perceived attitude, understanding or efforts. This could be considered a kind of *first order change*: a change that 'occurs within a given system that itself remains unchanged' (Watzlawick et al., p. 12). In this case, there was an expectation that the pupil would make changes to their own attitude or behaviour, whilst nothing else in the school system changed. This perpetuated the focus on presumed causes, rather than addressing the effects and interactions that occurred which could potentially lead to *second-order change*: a change 'whose occurrence changes the system itself' (p. 12), and therefore needs to involve those within that system. In education, this could be considered as the difference between attributing problems as situated within-child as compared to thinking about how the system around the child could change. Commonly, the intervention was regarded as a stepping-stone to something more desirable, such as Statement of Special Educational Need, reinforcing the construction of the EP role as a gatekeeper to resources.

Souter (2001) describes how '[i]n traditional approaches a lot of effort may be directed at one individual without success' (p. 39). In this school, arguably, change was taking place. Often these pupils were excluded, sent to a referral unit, or stopped attending. Sometimes this seemed to represent favourable change for the school system. Souter advocates moving away from models of linear causality towards an investigation of how the problem is reinforced by the actions of others within the system in a circular way. The implication of this, of course, was that I had to think of the pressures and expectations being placed upon the school system by other relevant systems such as the local authority – some of my work dialogue, therefore, needed to be redirected accordingly. I also discovered that the school did not perceive any value in making staff available to engage in consultation with the EP, and instead preferred the idea of the EP working directly with the child. 'But to achieve what?' was the question in my head. Systemic consultation was a way of working that I ultimately desired. I felt tied by the constraints of the context in which I worked, including that of employee of a local education authority where there were expectations of my role in helping to classify children's needs from a 'within-child' perspective through the process of statutory assessment. Yet at other times in my casework I was trying to present an alternative message. I wondered if this meant that my methods and intentions were unclear, maybe at times contradictory, and how this could also contribute to the homeostasis I felt so keenly. I found myself reflecting on McNamee's (1996) work a great deal. She frames the issues I describe within the concept of the construction of identities. For example, when discussing the *Diagnostic and Statistical Manual of Mental Disorders* (American Psychiatric Association, 2013), McNamee proposed that the use of such definitive guidelines placed those in the position of mental distress as 'objects to be studied, classified, and subsequently treated' (1996, p. 147). This was an observation that aligned with my own concerns. McNamee further explained that stories as told by these individuals, in this case secondary school pupils, are not enacted in the hope of co-constructing new narratives as may happen within therapy, but are instead 'heard as evidences of relatively enduring features of personal character in need of cure, adjustment, re-alignment or fine tuning' (p. 7). Here I felt positioned (Harré et al., 2009) as the 'fine tuner', engaged in a process which had the potential to reinforce this view.

There were times of hope and opportunity, however, such as when I stumbled upon allies within the school system. These allies, as I thought of them, tended to be staff who could see things from a different perspective, who recognised the value in a systemic dialogue. I thought of Winslade and Monk's (2007) ideas that the very complexity of the secondary school system can also be reframed as the very real potential for diversity within the members of the system (the staff, the managers, the pupils, the volunteers), which provides an opportunity for helping the pupil by working directly with the community of people around that pupil. As Winslade and Monk explain, it renders 'more likely the existence somewhere in the school of a "community of acknowledgement" for each person's struggle' (p. 130). This certainly seemed so. The work with school staff, in thinking about the needs of these pupils, became an opportunity to reframe the role of the psychologist as not an expert diagnosing problems but as a professional who was co-explorer in a process of meaning-making within a system. It became an opportunity to invite people into a dialogue, a relational exploration. It became an opportunity to very gently begin the process of change, allowing the ripples across the surface of such systems to gradually take on a life of their own.

Working systemically within special schools (Amy Hamilton)

Being systemically minded is something of an essential requirement when working to support the needs of children and young people with learning disabilities within an educational context. Throughout their lives, and before being referred to an EP, each child and young person with a learning disability has been on a journey usually involving several professional agencies (Keen, 2007). Each child or young person has their own unique needs which vary in severity and complexity and which change constantly over time and place. In addition to all of this, each child or young person exists within their own family circumstances, with parents who have experienced their child's journey first hand and have their own story to tell. In some cases, more commonly than I might have anticipated prior to entering the profession, families may have more than one child with a learning disability which can contribute a further layer of complexity, both practically and emotionally. After considering all of this, there are an additional number of practical elements that also need to be thought about: the type of provision which the child or young person with a learning disability is likely to attend and any transport arrangements, respite support, family support and extra-curricular activities they access.

As an educational psychologist, when a child or young person with a learning disability is referred to me, it is more often than not because of some concern held by the school or family (or both) for their well-being (e.g.

their behaviour has deteriorated or they have stopped responding to familiar routines in their typical way). Given the specialist nature of the services
a child or young person with a learning disability is often involved with, and
the knowledge and skills held by the adults around them, there has often
already been a round of 'troubleshooting' to little avail and they are looking
for something 'more' or 'different' from the EP. Through my practice in special schools, it often seemed that parents, professionals and school staff work
in silos, each trying to manage the situation in their own way with little to no
collaboration. I have often wondered what the many reasons for this might
be: professional remits, parental exhaustion, professional burn-out, parental disempowerment, school time and resourcing pressures, or perhaps the
potential for the dominance of reductionist views concerning highly context-
specific parental or school influence in the difficulties of pupils (Christenson &
Reschly, 2009).

As already noted within this chapter, systemic practice is something that
is embedded within many frameworks of educational psychology practice.
Arguably, this has been increasingly evident since the 1970s where the profession of educational psychology dramatically shifted its applied focus to
acknowledge that 'the social systems and organisations in education were
the more appropriate focus for psychological intervention than the individual
child' (Kelly, 2008, p. 21). Above, I have outlined the various complexities and
considerations that should be taken into account when working with children
and young people with learning disabilities, even if the 'problem' is apparently 'only' school based. To accept a referral with a view to assessing the
child in isolation and forwarding on recommendations to parents and school
in the form of a report would be naïve and unhelpful, and would most likely
lead to frustrations for the recipient (e.g. 'X won't work because the author
has not considered Y', and 'that recommendation has already been tried'),
further disenfranchising them and missing opportunities for collaborative
change. There is so much richness and understanding of the child's needs to
be elicited from those people already involved. Through collaboration, it is
possible to explore and enable change in the systems around the child, which
is so often where the issues are arising from (Every Child Matters, DfES, 2003;
Wagner, 2008).

Whilst I utilised EP consultation skills (including systemic thinking) in my
practice with special schools, I often found that a one-hour consultation
was never enough to hear the stories, the complexities and the wonder-
ings and to piece this all together in a collaborative and meaningful way to
promote positive change. Wagner (2008) describes how this consultation
approach adopted by EPs 'provides time and space for busy professionals,
such as teachers, etc.' (p. 148). She proposes that a consultation between
an EP, school staff and parents should last between 45 minutes and one hour
(Wagner, 1995). There is an element that the amount of time and space

allowed is dependent upon the systemic pressures that continue to ensure that all professionals in education are 'busy', but perhaps at the expense of truly giving time and space to focus upon children and young people with learning difficulties. There is a clear tension here associated with the time required to adopt a truly collaborative position, which once again highlights differences between first- and second-order approaches as described by Pelligrini (2009), where second-order approaches 'reject the "first order" expert position, in favour of a "collaborative not-knowing position", which engages clients in therapeutic conversations and facilitates the co-construction of alternative meanings about clients' lives' (p. 273). Further, time constraints risk placing professionals within an expert role, which can align with the expectations that parents may hold about professionals involved with young people with learning difficulties, and this then becomes negatively reinforced in a circular way. For example, in one school, working in silos had become so much the norm that little home–school collaboration happened, and when it did parents seemed disempowered and passive in the process of working with the school to enable change or voice their concerns. This perspective was later shared in discussion with a clinical psychologist who also worked in the school and prompted us to agree to approach the school's head teacher and share our thoughts. Through discussion with senior staff, it seemed that this was just a culture that had emerged over time through changes in management and so forth. However, greater home–school–professional collaboration and parental empowerment was something that they were keen to achieve.

The outcome of these conversations was the Family Space project, a joint project led by me as the school's EP, and a clinical psychologist. The project adopted the basic model of 'network training' which is utilised frequently within the field of learning disabilities (Jenkins & Parry, 2006). The aim was, and remains, to provide the opportunity for parents to self-refer to a Family Space meeting, hosted by both psychologists, with representation from school (including senior leadership and classroom staff) and any other professionals involved. Parents are encouraged to bring along family members for support but also for their insights. The meetings can last for up to three hours, with time for breaks. There is a more informal approach than in most school-based meetings, although we follow a general structure. We recognise that there are some potential challenges in relation to these meetings being held within schools, as maybe this implies a power imbalance, but at the heart of the idea is the hope that it situates the school at the centre of the child or young person's community. The meetings encourage everyone to share their views and to ensure that all views are held equally. There is time given to collaborative formulation around the co-constructed 'key change issue'. The model of formulation is selected according to the issue being discussed and led by the psychologists (e.g. functional behavioural analysis or cognitive-behavioural approaches). Towards the end of the Family Space meeting, time is offered to encourage reflection through the use of reflective circles (Schon, 1991). The reflective circle is created by placing two circles of chairs on either side of the room. The first circle includes family members, school staff and other professionals and the second circle includes the psychologists. The reflective circle with family and professionals takes some time and space to reflect aloud on the process, current thinking and ideas to take forward whilst the psychologists in the second circle take the time to listen. After this, the psychologist's circle is used as a space to reflect aloud on positive efforts, relationships and thinking as well as to acknowledge continuing tensions. The use of reflective circles is very powerful in 'bringing together' the system after much fragmented discussion. Although in its infancy, the use of the Family Space project to increase systemic and collaborative dialogue within a special school has been well received.

Conclusion

As different educational professionals we have each offered our perspectives, rather than answers, on the value and challenges of systemic working. In exploring the questions posed at the beginning of this chapter a number of common threads have emerged.

Why do we want to work this way?

Systemic practice allows us to positively position ourselves and be aware of the relational aspects of the complex and multiple systems within education. It allows us to challenge the traditional and more linear approaches, enabling us to distance ourselves from what we perceive to be an unhelpful within-child focus.

How are we trying to do this?

Even in creating this chapter we notice differences in the application of our systemic ideas. There is more than one way to be a systemic practitioner in education; we are doing it differently from each other. We try to apply systemic thinking and working by facilitating a collaborative and respectful way of working, maintaining curiosity, valuing and including the voices of stakeholders equally. We are also challenging more traditional beliefs about time and what is constructed as 'useful'.

What makes it difficult?

Difficulties we experience in working this way include perceptions held of our role (for instance, as linear practitioners and gatekeepers to resources) and the processes in the systems which reinforce those perceptions. In order to try to apply systemic working in the complex systems within education a level of energy and perseverance is needed, as well as maintaining an alliance with like-minded colleagues. This can be a challenge at times.

Who benefits from this approach?

All the stakeholders, through developing shared understandings of what constitutes the 'problem'. Systemic practice offers opportunities to reframe a limiting within-child focus as one which is located within the systems (education, family, community) around the child. As practitioners, there is a level of authenticity to being systemic: it's a better fit with our professional values as psychologists, where the contributions of those influencing the systems are respected and valued equally. In embracing multiple systems, we hope to create opportunities for mutually beneficial ways of working.

References

American Psychiatric Association. (2013). *Diagnostic and Statistical Manual of Mental Disorders*, 5th ed. Arlington, VA: American Psychiatric Publishing.

Christenson, S.L. & Reschly, A.L. (2009). (eds) *Handbook of School-Family Partnerships*. New York: Routledge.

Department for Education and Skills (DfES). (2003). *Every Child Matters*. London: HMSO.

Draeby, I. (1995). To see the world anew. In D. Campbell, *Learning Consultation: A Systemic Framework* (pp. 113–122). London: Karnac.

Fox, M. (2009). Working with systems and thinking systemically – Disentangling the crossed wires. *Educational Psychology in Practice*, 25(3), 247–258.

Freeman, J., Epston, D. & Lobovits, D. (1997). *Playful Approaches to Serious Problems: Narrative Therapy with Children and Their Families*. London: Norton.

Gameson, J., Rhydderch, G., Ellis, D. & Carroll, H.C.M. (2003). Constructing a flexible model of integrated professional practice part 1 – conceptual and theoretical issues. *Educational and Child Psychology*, 20(4), 96–115.

Harré, R., Moghaddam, F.M., Pilkerton-Cairnie, T., Rothbart, D. & Sabat, S.R. (2009). Recent advances in positioning theory. *Theory Psychology*, 19(5), 5–31.

Haselbo, G. & Nielsen, K.S. (2000). *Systems and Meaning: Consulting in Organisations*. London: Karnac.

Jenkins, R. & Parry, R. (2006). Working with the support network: Applying systemic practice in learning disabilities services. *British Journal of Learning Disabilities*, 34(2), 77–81.

Jones, E. (2003). Working with the 'self' of the therapist in consultation. *Human Systems: the Journal of Systemic Consultation and Management*, 14(1), 7–16.

Keen, D. (2007). Parents, families and partnerships: Issues and considerations. *International Journal of Disability, Development and Education*, 54(3), 1–18.

Kelly, B. (2008). Frameworks for practice in educational psychology: coherent perspectives for a Developing Profession. In B. Kelly, L. Woolfson & J. Boyle (eds), *Frameworks for Practice in Educational Psychology: A Textbook for Trainees and Practitioners* (pp. 15–30). London: Jessica Kingsley Publishers.

Mason, B. (1993). Towards positions of safe uncertainty. *Human Systems: The Journal of Systemic Consultation & Management*, 4, 189–200.

McNamee, S. (1996). Therapy and identity construction in a post-modern world. In D. Grodin & T.R. Lindlof (eds), *Constructing the Self in a Mediated World* (pp. 141–155). London: Sage Publications.

Moran, H. (2014). Using Personal Construct Psychology (PCP) in Practice with Children and Adolescents. https://issuu.com/pcpinpractice/docs/using_personal_construct_psychology (accessed 14 September 2018).

Newton, C., Taylor, G. & Wilson, D. (1996). Circles of Friends: An Inclusive Approach to Meeting Emotional and Behavioural Needs: *Educational Psychology in Practice*. https://inclusive-solutions.com/circles/circle-of-friends (accessed 14 September 2018).

Nolan, A. & Moreland, N. (2014). The process of psychological consultation. *Educational Psychology in Practice*, 30(1), 63–77.

Pelligrini, D.W. (2009). Applied systemic theory and educational psychology: Can the twain ever meet? *Educational Psychology in Practice*, 25(3), 271–286.

Rhodes, J. & Ajmal, Y. (1995). *Solution Focussed Thinking in Schools*. London: BT Press.

Schon, D.A. (1991). *The Reflective Practitioner: How Professionals Think in Action*. London: Taylor & Francis Publishing.

Souter, K. (2001). The relevance of systems theory for teachers dealing with emotional and behaviour problems in schools. *Pastoral Care in Education*, 19(1), 36–41.

United Nations (1989). The United Nations Convention on the Rights of the Child. https://www.unicef.org.uk/wp-content/uploads/2010/05/UNCRC_united_nations_convention_on_the_rights_of_the_child.pdf (accessed 8 January 2019).

Wagner, P. (1995). *School Consultation: Frameworks for the Practicing Educational Psychologist. A Handbook*. London: Kensington and Chelsea EPS.

Wagner, P. (2008). Consultation as a framework for practice. In B. Kelly, L. Woolfson & J. Boyle (eds), *Frameworks for Practice in Educational Psychology: A Textbook for Trainees and Practitioners* (pp. 139–161). London: Jessica Kingsley Publishers.

Watzlawick, P., Weakland, J.H. & Fisch, R. (1974). *Change: Principles of Problem Formation and Problem Resolution.* California: Norton Publishing.

Winslade, J. & Monk, G.D. (2007). *Narrative Counselling in Schools: Powerful and Brief.* London: Sage Publications.

9

Systemic Ideas and Positive Behaviour Support in a Crisis Service

Karin Fuchs and Peggy Ravoux

Accessible summary

- Positive Behaviour Support (PBS) is a way to support people with learning disabilities who show behaviour that can be described as challenging. It can work alongside other ways of helping people.

- Systemic approaches are often highly valued by families and networks. They help people find new ways to talk together so that they can find ways forward.

- Making the 'network of support' stronger through regular meetings and using systemic ideas called Open Dialogue can be very useful when people are in a crisis.

- In our service, families liked both the 'doing' approach of PBS and the opportunity to share and play a central part in their child's support by 'being with' and thinking about things with everyone together.

- PBS and Open Dialogue started from different ways of thinking, but both are about making sure that everyone has a part to play in making changes. This means it can be good to use PBS and Open Dialogue together.

Service context

We are clinical psychologists and systemic practitioners who have developed and led an enhanced intervention service (EIS) for adults with learning disabilities who display behaviour that can be described as challenging. The

EIS is a small multi-agency service which also includes nursing, social work, speech and language therapy and a behaviour support practitioner. The service was developed three years ago to help meet the Transforming Care agenda (Bubb Report, NHS England, Transforming Care and Commissioning Group, 2014) and support people with learning disabilities who display behaviours that challenge and are at most risk of placement/family home breakdown and/or hospital admissions locally, as well as complex people returning to area. We work in a diverse inner-city London borough, where a lot of our clients may be living with their families with complex support arrangements. The aims of the service are:

1. Crisis intervention: getting involved quickly and intensively at the point of crisis to assist in crisis management; intensive multi-element assessments; and intervention, training, support planning and care coordination.

2. Proactive work around helping design, develop and sustain 'capable environments' (Royal College of Psychiatrists et al., 2007) by ensuring local support arrangements provide a good fit with individuals' needs and supporting effective transition for people moving back to the area.

3. Working with identified local organisations, commissioners and other stakeholders to ensure local services are supported to work with a more complex cohort of individuals.

The service is positioned as an adjunct and/or additional intensity tier to the local community learning disability teams. More details on the Southwark EIS can be found in the 'Service Model Specifications' (NHS England, 2017).

In this chapter we explore the compatibility of Positive Behaviour Support and systemic approaches when working with people with learning disabilities presenting with behaviour described as challenging. We will outline how we use both approaches in our work within the EIS and in particular the positive contributions that systemic ideas and practice can offer within a crisis context. We will illustrate the model of working we have used in the EIS service with examples of our work and feedback we have had from families. Whilst the EIS is a small service, early indications from three years of data suggest the majority of service users with very complex needs have been able to be supported locally, with improvements in quality of life, reduction in challenging behaviour and positive feedback from families and other professionals. We try in this chapter to reflect on the added value of combining both PBS and systemic approaches to produce better outcomes for people. We also aim to reflect on some of the challenges and tensions raised.

Positive Behaviour Support

Positive Behaviour Support (PBS) combines the tools of behavioural intervention with person-centred approaches through multi-element interventions including functional assessment, skills teaching, behaviour support plans, staff training, modelling, functional communication, and Active Support at both a direct and organisational level (Allen, 2009). It aims to promote quality of life, enhance community inclusion and increase independent living skills, and is a person-centred and human rights-based approach. Assessment and formulation of the function of behaviours that challenge, within the individual's social and physical environment, are central to PBS (British Psychological Society, 2018). Whilst the evidence base is still growing, PBS is generally accepted and endorsed in policy, evidence-based guidance and professional guidance (Royal College of Psychiatrists et al., 2007; NICE, 2015; NHS England, 2017; British Psychological Society, 2018) and is also recommended as a key approach in reducing restrictive practice (Department of Health, 2014). It is therefore typically a cornerstone approach within service delivery for people with learning disabilities displaying behaviour that can be described as challenging.

PBS, like systemic practice, is an inclusive therapeutic model that works beyond an individual approach with consideration for the wider system. PBS as a framework involves the 'primary use of constructional principles and procedures from behaviour analysis to assess and support change' but includes the 'secondary use of other complementary, evidence-based approaches to support behaviour change at multiple levels of a system' (Positive Behavioural Support (PBS) Coalition UK, 2015). Likewise, there is consideration of engaging the wider system. At the centre of PBS, the engagement of stakeholders is central to the approach as part of the assessment and intervention with a focus on collaboration between clinicians and stakeholders. PBS can offer a clear framework for families and carers in terms of understanding how best to respond to behaviour that can be very challenging. We have found this approach very accessible to families and care providers as well as effective, and it remains a cornerstone approach within our model of service delivery. We have found that the PBS framework and systemic approaches are compatible and sit together well, and will describe in this chapter the added benefits of utilising both approaches in the context of an enhanced service working with people displaying significantly challenging behaviour.

Why integrate PBS and systemic approaches?

The idea of integrating PBS and systemic approaches is not new, but the evidence base around systemic approaches in supporting people presenting with challenging behaviour and/or combining systemic approaches with PBS is limited at present. Rhodes (2003) and Daynes et al. (2011) have explored the similarities and differences of the two approaches, arguing they can fit together well. We have built on this further, to compare and contrast these two approaches, as we see them, in Table 9.1.

The two approaches share some key similarities (i.e. considering the wider system) and both provide inclusive frameworks that can integrate with other approaches. Daynes et al. (2011) explore combining and augmenting PBS and systemic approaches in practice, for example highlighting when a behavioural formulation does not always 'fit' a family's perception of the problem,

Table 9.1   Comparing similarities and overlaps between systemic approaches and Positive Behaviour Support

	Positive Behaviour Support	Systemic Approaches
Focuses on understanding the meaning of behaviour	✓	✓
Intervention focuses on the wider system and environment	✓	✓
Considers the wider context of the behaviour	✓	✓
Focus of conversations (intention)	Problem focused with a view to promoting behaviour change and improving quality of life	Curiosity about multiple ideas, relationships and contexts, which can be wider than behaviour
Positioning of the clinician	As expert	Co-constructing and de-constructing of meaning
Epistemologies (theories or 'ways of knowing') of change	Behavioural, applied behavioural analysis	Relational, social constructionist
Culture and context	Contextual fit considered as part of intervention plan	Exploration of power and multiple contexts
Relationship to help	Not considered explicitly	Inclusive of patterns and relationships to help
Who is the client?	Individual, carers, services and organisation	Individual, family, system and organisation

Method	Assessment, formulation, functional analysis and multi-element intervention	Circular, relational, reflexive, exploring beliefs. Exploring multiple viewpoints, contexts and lesser heard narratives brings forth new ideas and potential for change
Outcome	Reduction in challenging behaviours and in restrictive practice; improvement in quality of life	Co-constructed outcomes whilst addressing risks and safety
Relationship to knowledge	Data-driven approach from a range of sources, objectivity	Multiple truths, use of reflecting teams and exploration of reflexivity

and show how creating therapeutic space with families can help them explore and share ideas and wider contexts in a different way and create more understanding of the space between families and clinicians. The position and the intention of the therapist is different: systemic approaches facilitate conversations with the aim of bringing forth multiple perspectives and potential ways forward; within the PBS framework, the practitioner, whilst working collaboratively with stakeholders, will offer an expert view. It is a more practical 'doing approach' in contrast to a 'being with'. Often when working with complex systems, particularly when families are closely involved or there are impasses in terms of change, a systemic approach alongside PBS can work well together, offering practical guidance alongside space to explore a more relational way of understanding and working with the network.

Systemic practice in the context of crisis for people presenting with behaviour that can challenge

Our context of practice is by definition one of crisis, related to complex clinical presentations associated with a significant increase in risks. The majority of people we work with are young adults, 17-and-a-half to 25 years old, living with families or hoping to move back closer to their families. There are often lots of people involved, and families and networks of support are often feeling quite desperate with support most likely on the verge of imminent or current breakdown. There may be pressing concerns about the client's immediate safety or their supporters' and younger siblings' welfare. There may be significant worries about what the immediate and long-term

future holds, and polarised ideas in the network about the best way forward. These aspects can significantly impact on the support network's
resources and capacity to engage in comprehensive clinical assessments at
the point of crisis. Families and services may already have developed discourses about each other and ways of working (or not) together, and often
there is a sense of an impasse. In the past they have often had limited input
from clinical services around behaviour and little experience of PBS, so
attempting to launch straight into, for example, functional assessments at
crisis point can feel too onerous and too different. We have found systemic
approaches very helpful to:

➤ Position families as experts.

➤ Help mobilise the network of support.

➤ Draw on and reconnect with their respective knowledge.

➤ Keep a relational focus.

➤ Help set a warm context for any PBS approaches.

Engaging 'stakeholders' or the network of support is key to both approaches,
yet in our experience in a highly charged context of crisis a more relational
approach within a complex network can be a helpful foundation to bind and
embed any future ideas in a way that feels within reach for the network of
concern.

We have found the Open Dialogue model, a systemically informed
way of working developed by Seikkula et al. (2003; also Seikkula &
Arnkil, 2006; Seikkula, 2015), particularly helpful in our work around crisis when used alongside PBS. This approach was developed in Finland as a
community-based crisis intervention for highly complex individuals experiencing an acute mental health crisis. The model has been evaluated over
a number of years and has demonstrated significant positive outcomes
on a range of measures including the prevention of psychiatric admissions (Seikkula & Arnkil, 2006; Seikkula, 2015). It involves mobilising the
support network at the point of crisis by facilitating regular meetings.
The engagement of families and supporters in the therapeutic process is
central to this approach and embedded from the beginning of the work. The
therapeutic conversations facilitated in the network meetings provide a safe
space to:

➤ Be listened to.

➤ Listen to multiple perspectives in the network.

➤ Co-develop meanings or try to make sense of things together.

➤ Share ideas going forward.

➤ Support the client *and* their family through the crisis.

Open Dialogue is an integrative approach to which other therapeutic modalities can be added or be offered alongside. In our context, this would be PBS, but also other multidisciplinary interventions, for example nursing, communication interventions and social care. The key elements of dialogic practice in Open Dialogue are a useful framework to illustrate how systemic practice can help and augment a more conventional PBS approach in our service context. We will therefore outline some of the key aspects of this approach (taken from Seikkula & Arnkil, 2006, pp. 51–128) which inform our practice, highlighting adaptations to working with adults with learning disabilities presenting with challenging behaviour, and connections with the PBS framework.

'Mobilising the network': Seikkula and Arnkil (2006) talk about the opening created by the crisis as a window of opportunity to mobilise the network by calling a meeting at the point of crisis. We find that a timely, flexible response at a point when the family and system most requires it is essential. We try and respond within 24 hours of having received the referral and from the start we introduce the idea of setting up an initial meeting for the network of support.

Burnham (2005) talks about the importance of relational reflexivity, and the different ways of warming the context of therapeutic invitation, coordinating resources by attending to language, emotionality and time in therapy. We have found this a helpful concept and the initial meeting and future network meetings are conducted as flexibly as needed and with a view to paving the way for our involvement. We take the lead from the client and their family about the timing and the location of these network meetings. We map out the support network and explore with the family and client who to invite, including who would be a resource to the client and the family. We explore how the adult with learning disabilities may be able to participate in' or contribute to the meeting and ways we can adapt our practice to ensure their inclusion, for example visual supports or dipping in to meetings, or investigating other ways their voice can be heard.

Box 9.1 Case study: Zara

Zara is an 18-year-old young woman of Nigerian descent with severe learning disability, and complex health and communication needs. She has a long-standing history of showing aggressive behaviours at home. More recently these behaviours have escalated to the point that they are placing a significant strain on the family relationships. The family had to resort to using emergency services and report being at breaking point. Zara's social worker is asking for our help to sustain Zara's placement at home.

▶

◄

We make contact with Zara and her family to set up an initial network meeting. The behaviour support practitioner meets with Zara and her family at home to get to know Zara. Zara's mother explains she wants the best for Zara and it is important she cares for her children at home. We ask who to invite to Zara's network meeting. Zara's mother suggests we invite Zara's grandmother and the family priest alongside her social worker and her key worker. We start the meeting by asking for Zara's hopes for the meeting: *'Getting a good plan together to help me be happy'*.

'**Social network perspective**': The network of support is invited to come together to work collaboratively as part of the crisis planning and intervention. Mobilising the system in this way, and quickly, sets a context for shared thinking and approaches to ways forward. In our experience it also galvanises the system and helps find energy and hope in the network for possible progress. As the conversations in network meetings unfold it may be that new people join these meetings at various points.

We invite the differing voices in the network to contribute to what *'Getting a good plan together to help Zara be happy'* would mean from Zara's perspective and hold onto some of the differences and similarities. We listen and acknowledge the dilemma and wish for *'a quick fix'* whilst recognising the complexity of Zara's needs and the family's situation. We start to hear the unspoken dilemma of Zara's mother, which the family's priest voices in one of the meetings: wanting the best for both Zara and her sister and what this means in the context of the family's culture. Gradually Zara's grandmother is able to voice her daughter's poignant realisation that she cannot continue to support Zara at home any longer. We start exploring alternative stories about what may be going on for Zara and her family and developing a shared plan going forward.

'**Taking responsibility**' and '**Tolerating uncertainty**': We take a lead in setting the meeting up, contacting attendees and warming the context for the meeting. We take responsibility for facilitating the meeting; however, there is no planned structure and clients/family/supporters are invited using open-ended questions to think about how they want to best use the meeting: *'How is it best to start?'* We ensure any ideas agreed as part of the conversation are shared promptly in writing and woven through the conversations as part of future meetings. It also creates a context and assurance around coordination and planning within the network of support. Families have told us that they valued the leadership provided as part of the coordination: *'It was like having a weight off my shoulders.'*

The type of therapeutic conversations in the network meetings and the focus on 'being with' and 'in the moment' serve a function of emotional containment for the support network. There is often a range of difficult emotions and experiences held by the network at crisis point. By inviting participants to share their views and experiences in the meetings, bearing witness and responding to what is shared by the support network, the capacity of the network to tolerate the unknown is strengthened. People are supported to put into words what may be difficult to name and their experience is validated, thus increasing their own resilience in the process.

Box 9.2 Quoting a parent: on being considered

'I was at rock bottom, the darkest place I have been since my journey with my son ... For me it was a godsend, they took over, chaired ... I was so overwhelmed as a parent in that place. You need someone to take the lead. I felt I was involved, they held my hand step by step all the way ... What about this, how about her ... how do we help her to help him? It was the first time someone was thinking about me'. (Parent)

'Dialogicity' and 'Polyphony': In the meetings conversations are facilitated to ensure everyone has a voice, is listened to and responded to. We ensure the perspective of the adult with learning disabilities who may not be present at the meeting or able to contribute to the meeting is held in mind by starting the meeting with: *'If A was here and able to tell us, what is it that he/she would want us to use the meeting for?'*

We invite attendees to take a listening position at various points in the meeting, drawing on the model of a reflecting team (Andersen, 1987) to share our thoughts and ensure everyone's voice is held in mind. The meeting room is a place where clinicians can also share their ideas, for example a PBS formulation or plan.

In a crisis context there can be huge pressure for an immediate solution, and attempting to carve out a reflective space and retain our own curiosity can be very difficult. It can also be very difficult at times when perceived risks run high to facilitate a genuine space where multiple perspectives can be heard and shared. The reflecting team creates an invitation for the network to listen to the team's thoughts and reflections as these encourage the support network to take a meta-perspective or 'birds-eye view' in a crisis where the capacity to think can often get lost. The network meetings set a context where it is possible to share and co-develop meanings about the crisis, and the person's and their supporters' strengths and resources. Through dialogue across the network of support new ideas can gradually emerge where it is possible to co-create alternative meanings and think about a way forward: *'a wonderful forum to share ideas, find solutions, share information and experiences of all.'* (Provider)

As psychologists in a small team, we tend to wear multiple hats e.g. care programme approach (CPA) coordinator, PBS practitioner, meeting facilitator, service lead and supervisor. Working alongside a PBS practitioner who contributes to meetings as an expert in their field is very helpful, as is having a trainee clinical psychologist on placement who can join us in systemic conversations. Capacity to respond in a timely manner to a crisis situation is often essential and in such contexts there are times when the boundary of our roles can become more fluid. We approach these situations by acknowledging the different levels of context (e.g. safety and risk, safeguarding, quality issues) which shape our positioning and the type of conversations we may need to have with people in the network. There are times when a higher order context may prevail, for example in the case of safeguarding or quality assurance concerns, and an expert position may be required. We reflect on the different positions we hold in a transparent way with the networks we have conversations with and reflect on these dilemmas as part of our weekly case discussions.

'Guaranteeing psychological continuity': As the meetings unfold, new narratives emerge about the 'crisis' and its meanings. Some of the conversations held in the network meetings can serve the function of information gathering from a multiple range of sources feeding into multi-element assessments, sharing formulations to date and co-developing reformulations with the network.

As professionals we can share our clinical dilemmas or suggestions of clinical interventions in a transparent way with the support network. The conversations held in the network meetings also feed into the development and review of the person's multidisciplinary care plan. Feedback from these assessments and any new information will be shared in these network meetings in a transparent way, so that the support network can explore together new meanings and ideas. The support network develops a shared understanding of everyone's role in the network, and shared goals and joint action plans supporting the client and their family. Families told us that they value the sense of accountability that the meetings were providing, thus conveying a sense of integrated working, continuity and progress.

The reflections and learning from the network on the crisis can inform future preventative strategies, which shape further the person's behaviour support plan.

Box 9.3 Case study: Lana

Lana is a 21-young woman of Ghanaian origin with a diagnosis of autism, learning disabilities and behaviours that challenge people and services. She has a history of placement breakdowns. Her current placement is breaking down. Lana's social worker is asking for our help to support her transition back to the area. There are multiple narratives in the support network about *'holding the truth'* about Lana's needs and the best way forward. We coordinate a series of network meetings to explore these multiple stories. Lana tells us she does not want to attend but would like her mother and sister to speak for her. We position the family at the centre and listen carefully to their story and experience of feeling disenfranchised in relation to services. We reflect on the range of experiences in the network supporting Lana and the richness of these *'multiple truths'* to set a context where it becomes possible to think together and co-create a shared vision of what *'good looks like'* for Lana's future support.

We have found using this plurality of approaches can really complement and enhance positive outcomes. The systemic approach enables a mobilisation of resources, engagement and coordination, an emotional therapeutic space and an opportunity for new possibilities that can feel very 'outside the box' but workable to the network of support that can go beyond 'traditional' solutions. It helps set up and warm the context for any future work and the continuity of work. PBS, however, can offer structure, focus on 'what to do' and assurance around safe effective practice that complements and feels necessary for supporting someone with such complex challenging behaviour, supporting someone with complex challenging behaviour in a crisis context. PBS practitioners in the team often have an added level of understanding of the system through the network meetings that is woven into their work with service users, families and carers.

Reflections and challenges

The service was born out of both the Transforming Care agenda and recognition locally that an enhanced clinical team could help avoid hospital admissions and people going out of area at a point of crisis. Whilst there was close interest in the potential outcomes, there was also recognition that the people referred, and their families and situational contexts, were complex. Often a PBS-only approach did not always feel a good fit with families and the new service and remit brought with it an opportunity to try out new models of working. We feel integrating PBS and systemic approaches has been key in the positive outcomes and feedback collated to date within the service. Families have consistently fed back that they felt central to the process and very much listened to. Functional assessments, the way reports are written, behaviour support plans, training and modelling would all clearly be recognisable considerations within a PBS framework and have been valued by families and the wider support system.

However, alongside a multi-element PBS approach, new and at times unexpected ideas have emerged via support network meetings, utilising more systemic conversations. These ideas will often come from families and be 'outside the box' solutions, but nevertheless central to a way forward. When reaching an impasse or when there is a sense of stuckness in the network these systemic conversations enable the exploration of narratives and new ways of understanding. For example exploring stories about caregiving and what it means in the family context may open possibilities and pave the way for solutions which may have otherwise been difficult to entertain, such as the provision of care outside the family home. Furthermore, systemic conversations held in network meetings are fundamental to enabling a context for the PBS and multidisciplinary teamwork by bringing people together, sharing experiences, discussing ways forward and agreeing the next steps.

Family involvement is embedded in all elements of the service. Families have been keen to maintain a relationship with us and update us on their journey post discharge. Families have been a key part of service development through participation in focus groups and co-production of videos with the intention of being helpful to other families and professionals by sharing their stories. We think that the way we position families and clients as expert by experience is central to this service development.

We have described how systemic and PBS approaches can complement each other, but there are times when families will prefer one or other approach and we have ensured we are responsive to that. For example, a parent listened carefully to our first reflecting team discussion and replied that it was a good summary, but could we get on with the action plan!

Whilst PBS and systemic approaches have very different language and epistemology, they both work with the system and both are approaches which describe themselves as compatible with other approaches. In our view it is not always a neat marriage but it can be hugely beneficial in engaging complex systems and making a more structured PBS approach more workable.

References

Allen, D. (2009). Positive behavioural support as a service system for people with challenging behaviour. *Psychiatry*, 8(10), 408–412.

Andersen, T. (1987). The reflecting team: Dialogue and meta-dialogue in clinical work. *Family Process*, 26, 415–428.

British Psychological Society. (2018). *Positive Behaviour Support (PBS): Committee Working Group Position Statement.* Leicester: The British Psychological Society.

Burnham, J. (2005). Relational reflexivity: A tool for socially constructing therapeutic relationships. In C. Flaskas, B. Mason & A. Perlesz (eds), *The Space Between: Experience, Context, and Process in the Therapeutic Relationship* (pp. 1–18). London: Karnac.

Daynes, S., Doswell, S., Gregory, N., Haydon-Laurelut, M. & Millett, E. (2011). Emergent Cake: A plurality of systemic practices. *Context,* April, 21–25.

Department of Health. (2014). *Positive and Proactive Care: Reducing the Need for Restrictive Interventions.* London: Department of Health.

NHS England (2017). *Transforming Care: Model Service Specifications: Supporting Implementation of the Service Model.* London: NHS England.

NHS England, Transforming Care and Commissioning Group. (2014). *Winterbourne View: Time for Change (The Bubb Report).* London: NHS England.

NICE (2015). *Challenging Behaviour and Learning Disabilities: Prevention and Interventions for People with Learning Disabilities Whose Behaviour Challenges* (NG11). Retrieved from: www.nice.org.uk/guidance/ng11 (accessed 14 December 2018).

Positive Behavioural Support (PBS) Coalition UK (May 2015). *Positive Behavioural Support: a competence framework.* https://www.skillsforcare.org.uk/Document-library/Skills/People-whose-behaviour-challenges/Positive-Behavioural-Support-Competence-Framework.pdf (accessed 14 December 2018).

Rhodes, P. (2003). Behavioral and family system interventions in developmental disability: Towards a contemporary and integrative approach. *Journal of Intellectual & Developmental Disability,* 28, 51–64.

Royal College of Psychiatrists, British Psychological Society, Royal College of Speech and Language Therapists (2007). *Challenging Behaviour: A Unified Approach (CR144).* London: Royal College of Psychiatrists.

Seikkula, J. (2015). Open Dialogues with clients with mental health problems and their families. *Context,* 138, 2–6.

Seikkula, J. & Arnkil, T.E. (2006). *Dialogical Meetings in Social Networks.* London: Karnac Books.

Seikkula, J., Aaltonen, J., Rasinkangas, A., Alakare, B., Holma, J. & Lehtinen, V. (2003). Open Dialogue approach: Treatment principles and preliminary results of a two-year follow-up on first episode schizophrenia. *Ethical and Human Sciences and Services,* 5(3), 163–182.

10

Working Systemically with Multidisciplinary Teams

Caley Hill and Cathy Harding

Accessible summary

- This chapter talks about using ideas from systemic theory to help teams support someone with a learning disability.

- The team might include the person's family, day centre staff, house staff, their community nurse, social worker, psychologist or other people who provide support.

- We talk about different stories team members might tell themselves to understand or make sense of someone's behaviour.

- Caley and Cathy talk together about different ways we can try and help teams to think about the stories they tell.

- We do this because stories can be changed and perhaps this can lead to teams doing things differently. Some ways to try and change stories are talked about.

- In the chapter, we think about how stories link to ideas about power, responsibility, what causes problems, and independence.

Setting the scene

Haley (1975) paradoxically outlines why systemic approaches are doomed to fail in teams, and Purdy (2012) discusses why they are not helpful in work with people with learning disability. They reflect on the grip that diagnosis, power hierarchies and individualised theories of causation have which can serve to reinforce problem-saturated narratives of distress being located in an individual and the importance of objective expertise in relieving this. Systemic approaches have challenged these ideas and propose viewing (often) complex systems around an individual with a learning disability as the client, in order to facilitate more hopeful resource-oriented conversations (Purdy, 2012).

Based on these ideas, we have been playing, experimenting with and refining systemic ideas in our respective teams for over a decade, with various degrees of success and failure. The chapter will focus on those that we have found to be helpful, with a nod to challenges we have faced.

We will outline specific methods which can be used at different points of the traditional clinical cycle, including: consultation; facilitating the individual's voice within teams; case workshops; the Tree of Life; and team formulation. Finally, we discuss our systemic ideas for working with teams when the team itself is having a difficulty. The chapter touches on hypothesising, neutrality and the importance of narratives.

A chapter in conversation?

Caley: Why have we chosen to narrate this chapter in conversation?

Cathy: Because it reflects how we usually construct our thoughts about the work we do and how we bring systemic ideas into our practice. Also, by talking together, we take the pressure off us as individuals to be an expert and allow the reader to see how we have constructed what we know, with the intention of being transparent. The footnote, however, is that we have edited it slightly in order to help it flow, for example adding headings, so that people can find their place and because we didn't speak in **bold** or with citations!

Narratives within our teams

Caley: I work in the NHS in a multidisciplinary learning disabilities team with a number of professionals including occupational therapists (OTs), psychiatrists, learning disability nurses, clinical psychologists and speech and language therapists. We are co-located with social services.

Cathy: I work for a small supported living provider. We have a clinical team of psychologists, OT and behaviour specialists. Our teams are only one part of the system and interface with people (services and individuals) that provide direct care for adults with a learning disability, both in the community and on inpatient wards: family members, paid carers, advocates, voluntary workers, friends and others who support the person on a daily, weekly or more ad hoc basis.

Caley: Some of the dominant stories my team tell are about how important it is that we have something to offer that is recognised as being useful, particularly at points of crisis.

Cathy: An important story in my team is that we have to both be independent and strive to always be better. There is also a narrative that we are criticised for being either too independent or not independent enough.

Caley: The stories we tell ourselves as a team are important, as they influence the meaning that we attribute to our own and others' behaviour. This, in turn, affects responses (Heider, 1958). The stories can be both positive and negative and include:

➤ Power: that the team has the expertise and resources to change things, which makes it frustrating when things do not change for the better. A risk with this story is that others, including the person with a learning disability, can be powerless.

➤ Responsibility: that the team is responsible for success and others are responsible for failure. This can serve a protective function for the team in that it does not need to look to its own role in contributing to failure.

➤ Causation: that challenging behaviour is a social communication, and if we understand what is being communicated then the challenging behaviour will alter.

➤ Dependence and independence: there are dominant cultural and professional narratives that a person with a learning disability needs to be working towards independence (rather than the interdependence that most people experience).

Our experience is that these narratives can become more dominant at points of crisis for individuals.

Cathy: Stories are always powerful if they are treated as if they are truths.

Systemic consultation

Caley: OK, so let's look at initial consultation. When we receive a referral, we invite the referrer to come and talk to us.

Cathy: It's the first opportunity we have to use systemic approaches when referrals are made to us as the clinical psychologists in the team.

Caley: What I've noticed about how these consultations have changed over time is that now I will have a much longer period where we have problem-free talk. I think this is related to my becoming more confident about not being 'expert' or solely responsible for solutions. Also, consultees have positively engaged, with more time spent talking about the individual, their stories, and their context, which has led to multiple shared hypotheses being developed. This 'feedback' has positively reinforced the change in how I position myself in consultations.

I tend to start by asking about the individual with the learning disability and their personality and temperament. From this I ask about other stakeholders in the system around the person. I usually do this by constructing a genogram. I ask lots of questions about the stories that are told in this system, using the GRRAACCES model (Burnham, 1993) to ensure that I incorporate a wide range of aspects of diversity. For example, what are the gender scripts in this family? I explore whether there are patterns of relationships over the generations. For example: 'Do mothers and daughters have conflictual relationships?' 'Are fathers absent?' I hold in mind how the system has adapted at life cycle transitions (Hayley, 1973; Carter & McGoldrick, 1980, 1989). Using the cultural genogram model (Hardy & Laszloffy, 1995), I ask questions about pride and shame issues for the system: 'Who are the decision makers?' 'What is the power hierarchy in the system?' Nearer the end of the session I will start to ask about the problem: 'Why is the referral being made now?' 'Who wants to change the most?' and 'Have individuals got any ideas about what will help?' I do this to try and understand the agenda and who might not want help. I will ask about each individual's relationship to help (Reder & Fredman, 1996). For example: 'What is the meaning of turning to professionals for help for this family?' 'What are the stories told about help seeking?' 'What is a problem for whom?' 'What has been tried previously and what was useful?'

The consultation sessions are only for an hour, so the questions I ask by no means cover every area I'm interested in. I've mentioned the key areas I focus on. The first 50 minutes are problem-free talk. In this time, I don't offer any advice. My experience has been that there is an element of interventive interviewing (Tomm, 1987), in that I invite the people in the room to consider a relational and contextual understanding of why there are difficulties. As a result, the conversation serves not merely as a fact-finding interview but also as a first intervention to create difference and potential for change in the system.

The referrer and I spend the final 10 minutes developing circular (relational) hypotheses about why difficulties might have arisen and what might be maintaining them. Having said this, sometimes there are practical things that need to be explored. For example, physical health needs must always be considered when a client has non-verbal communication, to ensure that an urgent medical condition is not overlooked in favour of a relational hypothesis. The tragic case of Richard Handley who died in 2012 from the complications of constipation is just one example of this (please refer to Chapter 6 for a more in-depth discussion of the context of diagnoses).

At the end of the consultation, the referrer and I discuss next steps and there could be a range of possibilities. I've noticed that often when I ask my questions about relationships, values and context, the referrer often doesn't know the answer. This provides an opportunity to suggest getting people together, or to meet with individuals in the system, including the person with a learning disability, to find out more about their perspective.

Hypothesising with teams

Caley: Actually, I've just thought that I talked about hypothesising during the consultation but I think we should talk about what hypothesising looks like. Hypothesising and re-hypothesising happens at all stages of the clinical cycle. The prompt to re-hypothesise is when we receive feedback. This brings in the idea of circular hypotheses. I always refer back to Gregory Bateson (1972) in relation to this and his theory that person A influences person B, and B's response influences A. So the idea is that my actions influence you and your actions influence me. Thus the hypotheses are circular in that they take into account that people influence each other. The other thing I was going to say is that it felt really weird to me, at the beginning of my systemic journey, to be hypothesising on the basis of nothing as I saw it then: I was more comfortable waiting until I thought I knew what was going on. Using the systemic model means that you hypothesise even though there might be no evidence to support them. It relates to the concept that hypotheses are just ideas about what is happening between people. It's breaking that ice, just doing it, and it helps me to not get married to a particular idea (hypothesis). I think it's important to generate lots of hypotheses to maintain this openness.

Cathy: And one of the things that I've noticed about your hypothesising as well, is that it goes a long way. It's not just that A affects B affects A, but A affects B to C to D back to B, etc. It's not just about making a one-step relationship in your hypothesis. It's about following that hypothesis quite a long way so it's truly circular in that it takes into account multiple relational interactions.

Caley: I think what I'm trying to do is to acknowledge the complexity of the system given there are multiple stakeholders and therefore lots of relationships that influence each other. I probably over-complicate things at times.

Cathy: I think that it can be a really helpful thing to think about throughout the process. Hypothesising about what's keeping the difficulty going, taking into account all the different parts of the system and their relationship with each other. I wonder whether we should give some examples of these? Below are some tentative circular hypotheses about interactions we have observed between teams and other parts of an individual care system.

Box 10.1 Examples of hypotheses

Responding to crisis

A displays significant behaviour or distress... a team member, B feels like this is a crisis... B goes to numerous people C and D. All these individuals communicate to A's family that there is a crisis... This makes A's family feel they cannot cope so they report more difficulties, as now they know they cannot cope alone... B feels that the crisis is worsening so keeps increasing the level of support... circularity.

Accepting care

A family system (A) have committed their love and lifetime to looking after a child with a learning disability who may have profound needs (B). When a care team (C) come in 'as if' they can fix all the difficulties, this gives the message (unintentionally) that family A hasn't done a good enough job. A feel devalued by this and begin to set increasingly high standards for team C to meet – leaving team C feeling devalued but determined to 'fix' the problems even more... So they work even harder and lead to family A feeling even more that they haven't done well enough... So the cycle continues.

Hearing the individual's voice in teamwork

Caley: So just touching on including the person with a learning disability's voice for a moment. We, or others, meet with the person with a learning disability to find out more about their perspective if possible and feed this into teamwork.

Cathy: Some would argue that valuing people and giving them a voice is the highest context marker within systemic approaches (e.g. Fredman, 2006).

Caley: Some of the systemic techniques we would use with a person with a learning disability to explore patterns of relationships, closeness, distance, issues of pride and shame, hopes, exceptions and resources include genograms (McGoldrick et al., 1999) or sculpting (Hearn & Lawrence, 1985).

Cathy: I might map Circles of Support (similar to Bronfenbrenner & Morris, 2006) with the person or complete a lifeline (Gramling & Carr, 2004) or a Tree of Life (Ncube, 2006). Other ideas might include video. This can be used to help an individual to prepare information to be shown to others within their network if they feel unable to share this directly.

Tree of Life

Cathy: So, one of the techniques I use, which aims to creatively use metaphor
          and story and externalise conversations, is the Tree of Life (Ncube,
          2006). It's centred on developing a life story and supports people to

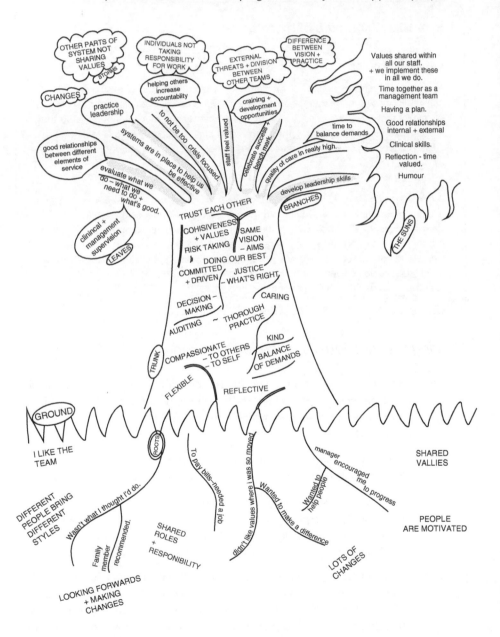

share these stories about their life; it externalises the conversations by allowing metaphor and playful elements to be introduced, with the aim of locating any difficulties as external to the individual. It allows difficulties to be seen as products of culture and history (Carey & Russell, 2004). It embeds many narrative therapy elements (Denbourgh, 2008) and supports individuals to think about their past, people who have influenced them in their lives, their key values, their strengths, hopes for the future and things that threatened these. I've used this with individuals with a learning disability (as in Baum & Shaw, 2015) and it can be helpful to share an individual's Tree of Life with teams (obviously with consent) as this allows the individual's views about their values and strengths to be seen, as well as how other elements, such as hopes and fears, influence their lives. It is one way to ensure the individual is held as central to team discussions, and that this is really the individual and not the problem.

Let's move on to talk about systemic techniques following referral and consultation to bring people together to have a shared discussion.

Case workshops

Cathy: Case workshops aim to bring the network supporting a service user together, to help the system work more effectively in supporting the person (Jenkins & Parry, 2006).

Caley: Some people won't know what we are referring to. They are often called 'network training days'.

Cathy: They were first referred to by Carr (1995) and Jenkins and Parry (2006). They are a way of inviting the system around an individual to come together (teams, family, carers, providers), usually for a whole day. It is often helpful to meet with the stakeholders to find out more information and expand opportunities for collaborative solutions. Questions are used to explore narratives in the system. This leads on to collaboratively developing hypotheses about why difficulties have arisen and why they are being maintained.

Caley: Why do we think it's relevant in learning disability multidisciplinary teams?

Cathy: Within learning disability services, as we have said, people might have large networks around them. They might be reliant on others for support in their daily lives and this is perhaps less likely to change. The advantages of having everyone together supports relatedness and creates connections in the network. It helps to see the priorities, struggles and dominant narratives of the different parts of the system in relation to, for example: power, causation, responsibility and interdependence.

Many of the discussions and questions and answers are recorded on flip charts, where possible with graphics. This is a way of making all the information group-owned and also ensuring that all the stories or ideas have equal value. These are then discussed and different elements weighted according to how they resonate with people.

Caley: I suppose now I think about it, the case workshops are similar to the initial consultation, with more people in the room, and it's a way of introducing systemic interventions. We might facilitate a workshop at the point of assessment, formulation, intervention or evaluation or repeatedly through this process. Case workshops provide a framework to elicit stories and encourage conversations and for people to share their ideas. We meet because a 'problem' has been identified. The agreed purpose is to develop some solutions but I would say my motivation is to increase stakeholders' options and opportunities to make choices about their lives and relationships.

In the workshop I will often start by developing some ground rules for the day with the participants, for example agreeing what is inappropriate and appropriate behaviour we expect of each other. Then we will map the system using a genogram of everyone in the system. We include ourselves in the genogram and acknowledge that we are part of the system and not neutral observers of it. This is often referred to as second-order cybernetics (Anderson & Goolishian, 1990). We are all full of strengths, assumptions, biases and vulnerabilities that we work hard to identify. We do this in order to remind ourselves that not everyone is like us, to open our curiosity (Cecchin, 1987) to other people's stories and reduce the risk of being blind to others or married to our own ideas. I hold the person with the learning disability in my head and encourage their voice to be heard if they are not present. Scaling (Berg & de Shazer, 1993) is another tool that can be used. I use scaling to elicit information, to draw out different perspectives, to gain feedback, and for evaluation. Scaling questions are asked, such as 'How bad is the problem now?' for different members of the system, and 'What could the best life look like?' Participants are then asked to rate (scale) their responses using numbers between 1 and 10, either individually or as a team, to elicit goals, track changes and identify differences of opinion between participants. This is summarised in Table 10.1.

Table 10.1   What to think about when setting up a workshop

Case workshops

Setting up a workshop

Invite as many people in the system as possible, think about venue able to accommodate this and how people who cannot be present might be able to contribute.

> **Ground rules**
>
> **Format** (what will be happening, emphasis on discussion and owned information)
>
> **Goals or aims** (this will include the opportunity to discuss/plan interventions to reflect on together. The idea is that this helps to open up the breadth of discussion not close down and solely focus on the problem)

The content

> What words describe the person?
>
> How the person spend their time/their likes and dislikes
>
> Who is important to the person and what are the support networks around the person?
>
> What are the key values of the family of origin that the person grew up in and how have these influenced members/how are they played out?
>
> What are the different temperaments of family/system members?
>
> How do different family/system members get their needs met or not?
>
> What are the stories that have been constructed about the Social GRRAACCES (Burnham, 1993) in this family?
>
> Whose voices are privileged and how?
>
> Whose voices are diminished, unheard or unrepresented and how?
>
> What are pride/shame issues in the family/system?
>
> What is the family's/care providers relationship to help?
>
> Are there any patterns in the relationships between people across generations?
>
> Exceptions, resources, noticing when the system does not engage in unhelpful patterns and why this is.

Cathy: As we've touched on, it's important to think about how the person with the learning disability can have a voice in the meeting if they aren't able to attend. Ways to do this include showing a video of the person talking about what they think is important, or to share their lifeline or Tree of Life. These same techniques can be helpful if the person does attend as well – they can present their tree, a lifeline or their own likes or dislikes (perhaps in a poster format). Again, individuals can make videos of themselves talking about these things, perhaps with someone they know well, and then show these in the workshop, as talking in front of a full room is a scary prospect!

Cathy: Towards the end of the workshop we encourage the participants to agree shared goals and develop multiple hypotheses and multiple solutions in order to help the group decide which of the hypotheses and interventions they are going to go with.

Caley: And do they get to decide that or do we decide that?

Cathy: They get to decide that!

Neutrality and truths

Cathy: Sometimes there are intervention ideas generated that we wouldn't go with, for example, if someone was to say we will punish an individual in response to certain behaviour. So, there are exceptions when I would say: 'That doesn't feel OK.' I would be quite transparent in this and say, 'I can't support this', but I would invite people to disagree with things that I might have come up with as well.

Caley: This is about the 'highest context marker' (Cronen & Pearce, 1985). What organises us and the boundaries we will not cross. I think the highest context marker is about safety and ensuring people are safe. Although you said earlier that for you it's the best possible care.

Cathy: And that would include people being safe!

Caley: Another one would be that we wouldn't act outside of the law, for example the Deprivation of Liberty Safeguards. Similarly, we wouldn't act outside our professional practice standards.

Cathy: In these situations, I don't maintain neutrality but I acknowledge sometimes these judgements are not clear-cut and are difficult to make.

Caley: So even though the stories we tell are just that, stories, some of these are truths to us as individuals and that is one of yours.

Cathy: Yes.

Box 10.2 Reflective questions on your highest context markers

- What are your highest context markers?
- What professional, personal, legal and ethical ideas organise your thinking and designate boundaries that you will not cross?
- Do the highest context markers differ when a person has a learning disability?
- Should they be different for different groups of people?
- What are the highest context markers for your colleagues or others in the system?

Team formulation

Cathy: Team formulation is another way of bringing a team together and having a conversation in relation to a problem. I tend to use this at the points of assessment and/or intervention. Overall, formulations aim to provide 'personal meaning and are constructed collaboratively with service users or teams' (DCP, 2011, p. 11). Systemically they relate very closely to hypothesising and feedback loops (see Vetere & Dallos, 2003, for a detailed explanation). The purpose of team formulation is to support the system to think about different perspectives regarding the 'problem'.

Primarily I've used the Nick Lake model of team formulation (Lake, 2008). It provides a framework that starts with developing a genogram and moves on to explore temperament, developmental history, cultural context, social environment when growing up and relationship history to stimulate thinking about relational expectations and ways of coping.

A genogram is a visual representation of a family or system that offers a tool that can be used across professional disciplines to record a family's stories, patterns and relationships (McGoldrick et al., 2008). It then uses the third element of the model to think about people's behavioural patterns, emotions and symptoms, as illustrated in Figure 10.1. I've used it with groups of between 5 and 20 staff to think about how the different elements influence each other using a co-constructive approach and enabling everyone to contribute to all the sections. This model draws on systemic theory as well as many other psychological and bio-psycho-social models. One of the reasons I think that this team formulation model is so useful is that it allows the team to experience safe uncertainty (Mason, 1993), to be guided to explore new concepts and ways to perceive difficulties. It does this in a safe way, as there are elements within the formulation cycle which are familiar (and therefore safe) for all practitioners, but it also allows the meaning staff attribute to a person's behaviour to emerge and ultimately impact upon how they support that individual (e.g. Ingham, 2011).

Team formulation allows us to develop circular hypotheses. For example, a person asks a staff member a question. The question makes the staff member anxious because they are worried that if they don't give the right response, it will result in 'challenging behaviour' from the person with a learning disability. So, staff respond in a way that they believe will reduce anxiety. For example, they give in and agree; but this leads the person to think 'I don't feel safe', 'I feel even more anxious', so they ask further questions and then everyone continues to go around this cycle, unintentionally keeping the problem going. So, I might ask, 'When the person does X, then what happens? Then what happens? And how does that feed back in to the behaviour being repeated?'

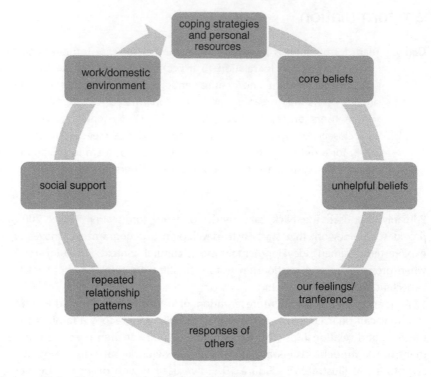

Figure 10.1   Team formulation (Lake, 2008, p. 21)

Caley: So, this illustrates second-order change, a change in meaning. In the example above, the staff member thinks the question means X but actually it means something different. Asking about how people respond to each other can lead to a new understanding of what the interactions mean to each individual. Thinking about what happens between people can present ideas for change as we come to understand how others interpret our behaviour. This approach also highlights how and why problems can emerge in relationships and be maintained (as opposed to problems being located in an individual).

Evaluation

Caley: Gregory Bateson (1972) noted that a system is any unit structured on feedback. This is the idea that systems change in response to feedback about the results of previous actions.

Cathy: So even though we use the format of the clinical cycle, we constantly invite, and try to be responsive to feedback. See Table 10.1 to see Lake's (2008) view of team formulation that reflects this approach.

Caley: I, very deliberately, set up interventions as 'experiments': 'let's see what happens', partly to mitigate some of the stories the teams tell themselves. For example, the story told about the importance of being experts, which can lead to a fear of getting it wrong. I also think it's important to try and foster a culture of accepting failure and emphasising that getting things wrong is OK. My other intention is to actively set up a framework to seek feedback, because we are interested in how it goes, and, if we need to change the intervention, hey that's no big deal – we didn't promise we would definitely get it right first time. In this, I have an intention of reassuring people that we are not perfect and get things wrong but it's OK, we can think again. This also opens up the option to jump back to the 'assessment' stage and use the clinical cycle of assessment, formulation, intervention, evaluation flexibly (DCP, 2011). The word 'experiment' is not used in a cavalier or disrespectful manner in this context and should not imply that ideas for intervention are developed casually or carelessly. Rather, my use of the term is based on the assumption that life is an experiment for all of us. None of us are so skilled that we can anticipate every outcome. The word is used to foster a spirit of hopefulness and willingness to try something different.

Cathy: Feedback can be sought in a number of ways, from formal measures to noticing comments that are made by members of the system after case workshops.

Caley: A really good way of getting feedback is when we invite the system back for a review case workshop. This allows us to gather feedback from a whole range of methods.

Working systemically when the team has a problem

Caley: What we mean by a problem is: when teams feel stuck or are split; when they are ready to give up; are in conflict; or have very different views.

Cathy: Some of the models we might use that we've spoken about are the Tree of Life (Ncube, 2006) or Team Formulation (e.g. Lake, 2008). These help the team to think how they and others connect. I've used the Tree of Life with teams to think about their team identity, either as individuals, then talking about the forest of life (Baum & Shaw, 2015), or as a team exercise, where the team work together on one tree.

Caley: So you use the Tree of Life to think about the team's response to an individual and as a way of the team thinking about itself and its needs?

Cathy: Yes, the model has been adapted slightly to focus more on professional identity (see Kis-Sines & Pluznick, 2014); this invites individuals to think about what led them into this work and why they wanted to work with people with a learning disability. It can also be completed by the full team working on one jointly constructed tree.

It can be helpful to the team to think about what the goals are of each team member and in relation to a specific situation. When people have different goals it can highlight why people are feeling dissatisfied. If everyone is working to a different end, then some people are not going to be happy with the outcomes that are reached.

Caley: Another idea that I sometimes use to inform my thinking when working with teams on their problems is a metaphor about whether doors to change are open or shut. Sometimes we push on doors that are closed, which can lead to getting stuck. Some of the techniques we've talked about (e.g. genograms and cultural genograms, McGoldrick et al., 2008), and particularly those questions which relate to people's relationship to help, can sometimes reveal that change is not sought or welcomed. It's often really helpful if this is identified so then attention can turn to what people can do given this constraint. Genograms or cultural genograms can also help people to see where they are stuck and where the openings for change are.

Cathy: When there are problems in teams, it can be very difficult to engage the full team. Sometimes this is because individuals within a team, even a systemically minded team, can fear their scripts being challenged and will not want to be part of team discussions. There might be established power hierarchies or established narratives about what produces change in others. When you bring people together to talk about an issue, it can be really helpful but also really challenging for people.

Caley: How do you work with this?

Cathy: It's helpful to ask teams to think about the dominant stories they are telling themselves about what they are good at, and not good at, and challenge some of these narratives. For example, I worked in a team where they were really good about telling stories where things had gone wrong and really bad at telling stories about what had gone right and made a really positive difference to people. Celebrating what's gone well helps conversations to not be entirely problem-saturated.

Conclusion

We have found it rewarding to use systemic approaches with teams. Teams have engaged with these ideas and they have led to positive change for individuals with a learning disability and other members of the system. This is in contrast to anecdotal stories that teams are notoriously stubborn when it comes to making changes to existing practice. We wonder if our experience shows that systemic approaches invite a genuine interest in team members' perspectives, validate and respect these and draw on their expertise and ideas when seeking to facilitate change, including their own experiences of negotiating challenges. Perhaps it is because we are mindful of the importance of being gradual in the change we bring and ensuring that we are respectful of the homeostasis of change. Or maybe it's because ideas are co-constructed and shaped by feedback, which reduces the pressure to get it right. This may mitigate a fear of failure by relieving a sense of individual responsibility or the need to hold an expert position and being solely responsible for success or failure. In our experience, teams are made up of people who are fascinated by stories.

The ideas referred to in this chapter have been used while simultaneously respecting Burnham's idea that a team 'must always remember that it will only survive if it is seen to be fulfilling the tasks of the agency in some way. If this factor is ignored, the team may be starved of referrals or less subtly disbanded' (1986, p. 73). In this context, using systemic techniques is not the priority; rather we have found them to be a helpful method in achieving our agency's highest context marker: supporting people with a learning disability to have fulfilling, meaningful lives.

If teams only ask problem-focused questions, they will only receive problem-related answers (Real, 1990). Using systemic interventions with teams allows narratives about power, responsibility, causation and interdependency to be explored. These narratives are present for people with a learning disability and teams at many levels. In our experience, if these stories are neglected there is a risk of unhelpful patterns of interacting with the wider systems which are so crucial to the lives of people with learning disabilities being strengthened and repeated, further thickening problem-saturated stories. Creating an opportunity for people to make sense of their relationships and context increases the freedom to enable stakeholders to make choices about their lives and relationships.

References

Anderson, H. & Goolishian, H.A. (1990). Beyond cybernetics: Comments on Atkinson and Heth's 'Further thoughts on second-order family therapy'. *Family Process*, 29(2), 157–163.

Bateson, G. (1972). *Steps to an Ecology of Mind: Mind and Nature*. New York: Ballantine Books.

Baum, S. & Shaw, H. (2015). The tree of life methodology used as a group intervention for people with learning disabilities. *The Bulletin*, 13, 14–18.

Berg, I.K. & de Shazer, S. (1993). Making numbers talk: Language in therapy. In S. Friedman (ed.), *The New Language of Change: Constructive Collaboration in Psychotherapy*, (pp. 5–24). New York: The Guilford Press.

Bronfenbrenner, U. & Morris, P.A. (2006). *The Bioecological Model of Human Development. Handbook of Child Psychology*. London: Wiley

Burnham, J. (1986). *Family Therapy*. London: Tavistock Publications.

Burnham, J. (1993). Systemic supervision: The evolution of reflexivity in the context of the supervisory relationship. *Human System*, 4, 349–381.

Carey, M. & Russell, S. (eds). (2004). Externalising – Commonly asked questions. *Narrative Therapy: Responding to Your Questions*. Adelaide: Dulwich Centre Publications.

Carr, A. (1995). *Positive Practice; a Step by Step Guide to Working Family Therapy*. Reading: Harwood Academic Publishers.

Carter, E. & McGoldrick, M. (eds). (1980). *The Family Life Cycle: A Framework for Family Therapy*. New York: Gardner Press.

Carter, E. & McGoldrick, M. (eds). (1989). *The Changing Family Life Cycle*. 2nd edition. Boston, MA: Allyn & Bacon.

Cecchin, G. (1987). Hypothesizing, circularity, and neutrality revisited: An invitation to curiosity. *Family Process*, 26, 405–413.

Cronen, V.E. & Pearce, W.B. (1985). Toward an explanation of how the Milan method works: An invitation to a systemic epistemology and the evolution of family systems. In D. Campbell & R. Draper (eds), *Applications of Systemic Family Therapy: The Milan Approach* (pp. 69–86). London: Grune and Stratton.

Denborough, D. (2008). *Collective Narrative Practice: Responding to Individuals, Groups and Communities Who Have Experienced Trauma*. Adelaide: Dulwich Centre Publications.

Division of Clinical Psychology. (2011). *Good Practice Guidelines in the Use of Psychological Formulation*. Leicester: British Psychological Society.

Fredman, G. (2006). Working systemically with intellectual disability: Why not? In S. Baum & H. Lynggaard (eds), *Intellectual Disabilities: A Systemic Approach* (pp. 1–21). London: Karnac.

Gramling, L.F. & Carr, R.L. (2004). *Lifelines: a Life History Methodology*. Retrieved from: www.ncbi.nlm.nih.gov/pubmed/15167509 (accessed February 2017).

Haley, J. (1973). *Uncommon Therapy: The Psychiatric Techniques of MH Erickson*. New York: Norton.

Haley, J. (1975) Why a mental health clinical should avoid family therapy. *Journal of Marriage and Family Counselling*, 1(1), 3–13.

Hardy, K. & Laszloffy, T. (1995). The cultural genogram: A key to training culturally competent family therapists. *Journal of Marital and Family Therapy*, 21(3), 227–237.

Hearn, J. & Lawrence, M. (1985). Family sculpting: 11: Some practical examples. *Journal of Family Therapy*, 7, 113–131.

Heider, F. (1958). *The Psychology of Interpersonal Relations*. New York: Wiley.

Ingham, B. (2011). Collaborative psychosocial case formulation development workshops: a case study with direct care staff, *Advances in Mental Health and Intellectual Disabilities*, 5(2), 9–15.

Jenkins, R. & Parry, R. (2006). Working with the support network. *British Journal of Learning Disabilities*, 34, 77–81.

Kis-Sines, N. & Pluznick, R. (2014). Tree of Life: Questions about professional identity for child and youth workers. https://dulwichcentre.com.au/wp-content/uploads/2014/01/tree-of-life-professional-identity.pdf (accessed 8 February 2017).

Lake, N. (2008) Developing skills in team consultation 2: A team formulation approach. *Clinical Forum*, 186, 18–24.

Mason, B. (1993). Towards positions of safe uncertainty in human systems. *The Journal of Systemic Consultation and Management*, 4, 189–200.

McGoldrick, M., Gerson, R. & Shellenberger, S. (1999). *Genograms: Assessment and Intervention*. New York: Norton Professional Books.

McGoldrick, M., Shellenberger, S. & Petry, S. (2008). *Genograms: Assessment and Intervention*. 3rd edition. New York: W.W. Norton & Company.

Ncube, N. (2006). The tree of life project. Using narrative ideas in work with vulnerable children in Southern Africa. *The International Journal of Narrative and Community Work*, 1, 3–16.

Purdy, L. (2012). How to fail as a family therapist working with adults with a learning disability: A paradoxical literature review. *Journal of Family Therapy*, 34, 419–430.

Real, T. (1990). The therapeutic use of self in constructionalist/systemic therapy. *Family Process*, 29(3), 255–272.

Reder, P. & Fredman, G. (1996). The relationship to help: Interacting beliefs about the treatment process. *Clinical Child Psychology and Psychiatry*, 1(3), 457–467.

Tomm, K. (1987). Interventive interviewing: Part II. Reflexive questioning as a means to enable self-healing. *Family Process*, 26(2), 167–183.

Vetere, A. & Dallos, R. (2003). *Working Systemically with Families; Formulation, Intervention and Evaluation*. London: Karnac.

11

Using Systemic Ideas in an Inpatient Setting

Esther Wilcox

Accessible summary

- I work in an 'Assessment and Treatment Unit' (ATU). An ATU is a psychiatric hospital unit adapted to meet the needs of people with more severe intellectual disabilities.

- People come to an ATU if they can't be supported in the community any more. This might be because they are very mentally unwell or if their behaviour is really challenging.

- People are usually admitted under a section of the Mental Health Act. This means they have been assessed as having a 'mental disorder' and needing to be admitted to hospital for their own or someone else's safety.

- The decisions made in ATUs have often been led by psychiatrists.

- Because of this, ATUs often understand 'the problem' mainly in terms of there being an 'illness' or other problem *in* the person that needs to be fixed (through, for example, medication, psychotherapy, or behaviour being controlled by staff).

- In this chapter I try to think about how systemic ideas can be used in an ATU setting and some of the challenges that might come up when trying to use them in a system which can have a very firm belief in the individual problems being in people.

I would guess that, for many people, the image that comes to mind when you think about a hospital is a very medical environment, a scrubbed place full of lots of specialised equipment, buzzing with nurses who are working under the direction of highly trained doctors who are applying science and logic (in a clear linear fashion) to enable the treatment and (hopefully!) cure of their patients. I work in a hospital ward but it's not really like this. The ward I work in is also known as an Assessment and Treatment Unit (ATU). The unit is within the NHS and offers support for adults with learning disabilities who are deemed to 'need' inpatient support and whose needs 'require' more specialised support.[1] People who are admitted usually have a more severe intellectual disability, meaning that their cognitive impairment is more notable than for someone who 'has' a mild learning disability, and the person may need substantial support in many areas of their life.[2] People have also often been displaying behaviours that their support system finds difficult – usually aggression to others, less often other behaviours such as being awake and extremely active for 20+ hours a day. Sometimes these challenges occur in the context of a severe mental illness. There are doctors (psychiatrists) and learning disability and mental health nurses working on the unit, but there are also support workers, psychologists, speech and language therapists, occupational therapists and physiotherapists. We work in partnership with social care colleagues, advocates and, of course, the person and their family. In this chapter I am going to talk a bit about how systemic thinking and ideas are relevant and useful when working in that kind of setting. I will start by telling you a bit about me, before saying something about what has been written in the past regarding systemic work in these contexts and then exploring how I use systemic ideas in my work.

My context

I am a white, British, female clinical psychologist. I've been qualified for 15 years and since qualifying (and for much of the time before) I have worked with adults with learning disabilities. For nine years I worked solely in community teams. I've been working mainly at the ATU for six years. Before training I had a few other jobs in the caring industry including with a social care team and a housing support team. A medical context is perhaps one which is reasonably comfortable for me. My mother, aunt and my father's second wife were all nurses. I spent time at the GP practice my mum worked at when I was a child. I also went to hospitals relatively frequently as a child, visiting mum after the operations she needed because of her arthritis and attending when I needed nebuliser treatment for my asthma. I am comfortable in a medical environment which is perhaps both a strength and weakness in my current role: I can function well in a hospital setting but may not always be well tuned in to how intimidating or uncomfortable the environment may be for others.

The service context

Systemic thinking reminds us that 'All behaviour makes sense in context' (Gehart, 2016, p. 54) and perhaps challenges us, therefore, to think 'in what context does this make sense?' when we come across things that seem odd or unusual. Thinking about the service context of an ATU might, therefore, help us to think about why it is as it is and therefore how we might use systemic ideas in a way that feels OK to those people working in and using the service. ATUs were developed as long-stay institutions were closing in the 1980s and 1990s. They were there to provide specialist hospital care when needed, though the idea was for the stays to be shorter term than the life-long 'homes' that the institutions offered. In many cases that has been the case, though there are also lots of people who have stayed in such units ever since the institutions closed and others who although they have had some experience of living in the community have spent very long periods of time in an ATU.

ATUs have rightly come under intense scrutiny since the Winterbourne View scandal of 2011 when undercover filming for the *Panorama* TV programme exposed widespread horrific and blatant abuse of patients in the Winterbourne View hospital (an ATU) by a number of nurses and support workers (www.bbc.co.uk/news/uk-england-bristol-20078999). The Transforming Care agenda in England that has resulted from this (www.england.nhs.uk/learning-disabilities/care) makes an explicit pledge to reduce inpatient admissions (the aim in the NHS's 2015 publication *Building the Right Support* was to reduce usage of such units by 50 per cent). Where admission to any such unit is being considered, the person's support team are expected to arrange a CTR (Care and Treatment Review – see www.england.nhs.uk/learning-disabilities/ctr). CTRs have a number of aims, including to 'prevent people being admitted unnecessarily into learning disability and mental health inpatient beds through identifying alternatives where appropriate' (NHS England, 2017, p. 13). It is impossible to very clearly outline exactly when admission is 'unnecessary', and this creates a context in which discourses of blame, responsibility and failure can become salient whenever a person is admitted to an ATU. Once blame is on the table, we know that an individual pathology discourse (i.e. saying that there is something wrong with the individual person, maybe in their brain or mental health) can serve to protect staff from blame but can also be disempowering for the person themselves (Wilcox et al., 2006).

Most people admitted to ATUs have been 'sectioned' under the Mental Health Act (MHA 1983 & Amendments 2007) which means they have been assessed as having a 'mental disorder' and as requiring inpatient admission because of the risks to their health or safety or risks to others (see the 2015

Mental Health Act Code of Practice published by the Department of Health if you want to find out more about the MHA and the criteria that need to be met before someone can be 'sectioned'). The MHA says that autism is a mental disorder, but that learning disability is not, unless it is associated with 'abnormally aggressive' or 'seriously irresponsible' conduct. The Act aims to protect rights and support ethical practice but also clearly creates a momentum pulling everyone towards constructing the person as someone who has a very clear 'individual pathology'. It is this that makes the admission possible, and necessitates that people who are free from such 'defects' must be the ones to sort things out. Most people who are sectioned need to allocated a 'responsible clinician' who must also be an 'approved clinician'. Other inpatients (e.g. people who have agreed to stay in the hospital) also need to have an approved clinician in charge of their assessment and treatment during their admission (Zigmond, 2014). To date, almost all approved clinicians, and therefore responsible clinicians, are psychiatrists. In recent years a small number of 'non-medical approved clinicians' have been approved and are working, therefore, as responsible clinicians (mainly, at present, psychologists). However, clearly at this point in time it is most likely that the person who is legally seen as the clinical leader for a person's care and treatment will be an experienced medical doctor.

These factors, I believe, can reinforce the idea that problems are located within the admitted client and that the purpose of an ATU is to ensure that experts can complete the right assessments in order to know what is wrong with the person and ensure that they are 'fixed' in the appropriate ways. The scrutiny which ATUs are under, together with the fact that the challenges which led to admission usually continue to present after admission, creates an incentive for the services to locate the problem within the person.

What have other people said about systemic thinking in ATUs?

Mason (1989) wrote about 'handovers' in residential and health settings (a 'handover' is what happens when the staff from one shift are leaving and the staff from another are starting work, with the aim of handing over relevant factual information, including how the ending shift progressed and the current status of the clients). He talked about how a number of systemic ideas could be used in settings which use 'handovers' (as is the case in the ATU in which I work), including a range of circular questions, and outlined a process for a systemic handover interview. However, there is a paucity of other publications which directly explore the use of systemic ideas in the ATU context.

Systemic ideas used in the Assessment and Treatment Unit

Working psychologically – and attempting to do that systemically – is a thought-provoking challenge in an ATU. There are occasions when I am working with a person who is staying in the unit, or their family members, in a 1:1 or family group context. Systemic ideas might need adapting to be more accessible for people with learning disabilities when they are used in this way, but there are no additional adaptations needed because someone is in an inpatient unit, though the context of admission will be borne in mind at all times (Baum and Lynggard's 2006 book is a great place to start to find out more about how to adapt therapeutic systemic approaches so that they are useful and inclusive when working with people with learning disabilities). Most of my work in the ATU is much less direct, however. A main source of systemic influence is through my attendance and chairing of the weekly to fortnightly 'ward round'-type meetings. These may be attended by the person, their family, staff from the health and social care community teams, and other professional supporters (including formal advocates or direct care staff from the person's home). Another key area for systemic influence is the multiple informal contacts I have with the support work and multidisciplinary team at the ATU on a daily basis. Below I will outline a composite case study and then talk about the ways that systemic ideas influence my work with the client.

Composite case study

So let's imagine a client (Josh) who has been admitted to an ATU and after that we can think about some systemic ideas and how they influenced the work with Josh.[3]

Josh is a 21-year-old man. He has brother who is three years older and a sister who is five years younger, all from the same parents who have been married for 26 years. He has been said to have a severe intellectual disability and severe autism. He has some verbal communication though does not initiate verbal interactions and will tend to answer any questions directed to him with single-word answers. Historical reports suggest that Josh's parents first sought help with his 'challenging behaviour', which included high-pitched screaming, smashing up household items and hitting others, when Josh was 7. Over the years the family has had a lot of contact with services. The challenging behaviours waxed and waned a little but continued to be seen regularly. Problems escalated as Josh got physically larger. Josh left the family home when he was 18 as the family felt they could no longer support him and keep everyone safe. He lived in four residential homes between the ages of 18 and 20 at which point he spent 12 months in another ATU. He moved into his fifth home when he left there at age 21. That placement lasted five months and the service struggled to support him throughout that time. Josh was frequently distressed and aggressive. Following a more serious assault on a member of staff, Josh was admitted to the ATU under Section 3 of the MHA (2007). At the point of admission he was taking very large doses of anti-psychotic medication (though he had no diagnosis of severe mental illness) and consequently found it very hard to stay awake during the day. When awake he was often aggressive towards the staff supporting him and sometimes towards other clients in the ATU. His parents and siblings were all highly stressed and worried about him. They had visited him regularly in all the places he had lived since leaving home and were finding it increasingly hard to see their son/brother so upset.

The difference that makes a difference and narrative ideas

Gregory Bateson coined the term 'a difference that makes a difference' (Bateson, 1972, p. 336) and for me this is a key thing to consider in all of my work at the ATU. If I try and introduce ideas which are too different from how the important people in the person's network (the person, their family, their community staff and the ATU staff, for example) are currently making sense of the world, then those ideas will fall on stony ground: they will not make a difference and people may think that psychology does not have much to offer, thereby reducing any potential for future influence. In order to try and have useful and sustainable influence, I have found that I need to understand and try to work alongside the dominant medical, individual pathology discourse but at the same time to introduce some difference to that thinking in order for the person's complete emotional experience and full personhood to also have space. Although I may hold in mind some of the erudite publications which offer a more radical examination of the current constructions of disability (see Haydon-Laurelut, 2015, for example) or mental illness (see Johnstone, 2000, for example), I may also choose not to explicitly share some of the ideas which are in my mind as I work to try and remain aware of how I and others are currently constructing reality (e.g. the dominant discourse in the ATU is of autism being a neurodevelopmental disability: ideas about it being social constructed are very different and sometimes too different to be useful to people). I often need to present in a more expert way than feels entirely natural for me, as holding a not-knowing position and a multitude of possible hypotheses in mind can sometimes be too different to the expert position which the ATU engenders. Sharing my own thinking at these times can undermine my own influence and paradoxically, therefore, my ability to support the team to hypothesise more broadly. I find it helpful to think about Wooffitt's (1992) work which offers an analysis of how people describe paranormal experiences and how an analysis of their talk can demonstrate how they try and ensure that they come across as a reasonable and sensible person rather than a crackpot (meaning that you are more likely to find their descriptions of their experiences convincing). I need to be wary about being seen as 'over-psychologising' (this is an actual description I have heard regarding a colleague's intervention).

One way of addressing this dilemma is not so much to try and introduce any difference but, using narrative therapy ideas, to look for the 'thin' stories (see Box 11.2) which are already present in the talk of the team as a whole (including the person and their family). All colleagues – family members as well as health and social care professionals – do, of course, have a richness in their talk about any person/problem/situation, and narrative therapy offers a number of ideas about how those stories can be thickened and developed. As an example, one of the thin stories often encountered in the ATU may be about people being 'attention seeking'. Making space for further exploration of the contexts of people's lives and histories can lead to thicker descriptions such as that the person is very sociable but has had lots of experiences of being left alone (and lonely) for long periods of time and now worries that this will happen again. Stories about the importance of human connection for all can also diminish the judgemental power of the 'insult' of 'attention seeking' and allow a more connected and nuanced problem-solving approach.

Box 11.1 Is narrative therapy systemic?

This is a controversial question! Personally I do conceptualise narrative therapy as systemic as it is concerned with the connections between people and the sense making that happens in conversations. See Hayward (2009) for a really useful discussion of this question (and a brief outline of some different versions of 'systemic' theory).

Box 11.2 Stories in narrative therapy

White and Epston (1990) suggest that only a fraction of what people experience can be 'storied' and expressed so there will always be a dominant story about a situation alongside other more hidden stories. Experience falling outside the dominant (or thicker) story can be given greater strength (thickness) using narrative ideas. The stories we tell about our life and experiences have a great deal of influence on the future (as well as our understanding of the past). Increasing the influence of thin stories can therefore be very powerful. If you are new to narrative therapy ideas, see http://dulwichcentre.com.au/what-is-narrative-therapy.

At admission, the dominant stories were individual pathology discourses. Josh had disabilities (autism and severe learning disability) which indicated sub-optimal functioning. 'This is why he is challenging.' 'He needs to be fixed or his behaviour managed.' In addition, 'His parents did not "manage him" – professional experts are needed.' Josh quickly started to form relationships with his staff, however, and alongside this 'deficit-focused' talk there were also comments (from ATU staff) about 'how awful it must have been for Josh to have to leave home': these enabled conversations about staff members' experiences of leaving the family home and a connecting with Josh on a more human and less staff–client level. Staff talked about how unsettling it would be for many people to live in five homes and two hospitals in a space of just three years and also talked about the importance of the relationships Josh had with his staff, as well as acknowledging that the multiple changes he experienced would have made it very hard for him to get to know people and to feel safe. Staff talked about Josh's emotional reaction to those experiences and some-times compared them to their own experiences which they saw as somewhat similar.

In my previous research I called this sort of talk the 'context discourse' (Wilcox et al., 2006) and suggested that its use opens up the possibility of greater empowerment and creates scope for more optimism about the future. The whole team (including the person and their family) can work together to think about the sort of context which will meet the person's needs in the future. I did not explicitly offer 'interventions' to create space to thicken such discourses (in a 1:1 or other therapeutic sense) but in the contexts described above I paid attention to these stories, gave them space and asked questions which allowed them to develop. The ideas influenced a Positive Behaviour Support (PBS) plan which was shared with all the staff (see Box 11.3). The aims of the plan included validating these important ideas about Josh's life and experiences. I talked with staff about times when Josh was not aggressive (especially if Josh was in a situation where people might have worried that aggression may show itself) as one way to open space for other stories (Freedman & Combs, 1996). We talked about how autism and learning disability impact on Josh and, by thickening the stories from diagnosis to individual meaning, attempted to construct an understanding which both acknowledged the real problems that Josh faced in life (Goodley, 2011, cited by Webb, 2014) and storied him as an active agent, a nuanced person rather than just a 'patient'.

Walther and Fox (2012, p. 12) state: 'If identity is understood to be a social and public achievement, rather than an intrinsic characteristic of a person, then it is even more powerful when these alternative identity claims are pub-licly acknowledged by people other than the therapist.' They talk about using 'outsider witnesses' (people not involved in the therapy but influential in the person's life) to hear the new stories. The fact that these conversations were held in multiple contexts and with multiple others created a kind of informal 'outsider witness' situation which could powerfully embed the alternative discourses and identities. In all of these conversations I monitored how my talk was being received by others. Was I being 'too different'? If verbal or non-verbal feedback suggested I was, I sought to move myself towards a better understanding of the contexts which were influencing the people I was interacting with in order to try and make space for conversations which were close enough to the person's existing constructions of reality (as I understood them) to be heard, but different enough to potentially make a difference in Josh's life.

Box 11.3 Positive Behaviour Support (PBS) and PBS plans

PBS is currently a big influence on services for people with learning disabilities. It is a model which believes that challenging behaviours happen for a reason and aims to find out that reason and then support the person to meet their needs in other ways (without using any aversive or punitive approaches). A PBS plan is a place where the reason is written down, along with information about how to prevent challenging behaviour and how to respond if the person does start to get stressed or challenging.

You can find more information about challenging behaviour at: www.challengingbehaviour.org.uk/about-us/about-challenging-behaviour/what-is-challenging-behaviour.html.

You can find more information about PBS and PBS plans at: www.challengingbehaviour.org.uk/learning-disability-files/03---Positive-Behaviour-Support-Planning-Part-3-web-2014.pdf.

The strange loop – achieve change without anything changing?

'Strange loops' as a theoretical idea sits within the 'reflexive inquiry' extension of Coordinated Management of Meaning (CMM) theory (see Oliver, 2004). CMM is a model of communication which is based on a social constructionist view of the world. The theory has lots of ideas about how communication is central in the creating of social realities. A central concept is that we do not just passively 'see' or 'uncover' reality. We create it when we talk and communicate together. Pearce and Cronen were the original proponents of CMM. They suggest that communicative acts are linked to a specific context, but also always in 'multiple levels of embedded contexts' such as the culture, self-identities and relationships of those who are communicating. They suggest that the levels of context all impact on the communication, but that the communication can also impact on the context (have a look at Chapter 17 of this book, Pearce, 2007, 2012; Cronen, 1994; or Holmgren, 2004 if you'd like to find out more about CMM). CMM suggests that the words we say make sense within certain contexts but also that the words we say form the context. Oliver (2004) states that we often use communications which involve significant 'polarising' (e.g. good/bad; right/ wrong) but this often 'simplifies in a way that does an injustice to the richness and possibility inherent in communication' (p. 131) and can give rise to a strange loop.

I have noticed that a strange loop can often come into play when someone is admitted to the ATU (see Figure 11.1). When a person is admitted, the community team professionals, the family and the person admitted have usually spent a *lot* of time and energy considering what is going on, thinking about what will help and trying different solutions to the problems. They often feel they have exhausted every reasonable option and indeed that if that were not the case, this could open up the possibility that they could be blamed for not having implemented the alternative solution (as admission can easily be discoursed as a failure). There are, of course, many reasons why people have focused on the options that have been tried. In my experience, most practitioners who support people with learning disabilities are highly committed, thoughtful and often pretty humble people who are usually guided by a very clear moral code within which they interpret the ever-increasing sets of guidance regarding how services should work and how they should protect vulnerable people's rights. This leads to a situation where a different outcome is wanted, but people do not want (or feel able) to do anything differently. The resulting strange loop is shown in Figure 11.1 – it's not experienced all in one instant but over time and in response to the current situation (so when things are believed to be going badly, the person is much

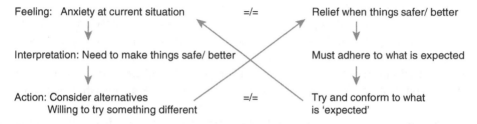

Organisational cultural story: Inpatient admission is a failure. Learning disability services are bad and disempower people.

Relationship story: It is my job to make sure others are supporting the person as we are told they should.

Identity story: If I had done things better admission would have been avoided.

Feeling: Anxiety at current situation　　　　=/=　　　　Relief when things safer/ better

Interpretation: Need to make things safe/ better　　　　Must adhere to what is expected

Action: Consider alternatives　　　　=/=　　　　Try and conform to what
　　　Willing to try something different　　　　　　　is 'expected'

Figure 11.1　Change without changing strange loop

more able to think about doing something 'outside the box' and challenging the sometimes limited ideas about what services should do, but when things are more stable then the person adheres more to the rigid ideas about what they 'should' do).

Oliver (2004) suggests that just identifying the strange loops we have become trapped in can be helpful. Changing the way we understand things at various levels of context can also help (e.g. changing/developing the organisational cultural story, relationship story or identity story).

The strange loop was very much in evidence during the conversations about Josh and his support needs. On some level there seemed to be a hope that he would be diagnosed with a severe mental illness, perhaps because then hopes could be pinned on a medication-related solution (and perhaps because such a step would absolve most of the team from blame). However, Josh's anti-psychotic medications were reduced and there were no indications that this increased his distress or led to presentations which could be usefully understood as a severe mental illness. The ATU team started to form some good relationships with Josh and noticed that he appeared more agitated when he was given lots of choice. The idea of valuing 'not overwhelming Josh' (an idea which ATU staff had developed) and offering more limited choice was mooted but these ideas did not fit for staff from the local community team who had been supporting Josh since adulthood and with whom ATU staff had generally formed reasonably positive relationships.

I hypothesised that we had entered a strange loop. There are many national drivers (organisational contexts) which highlight the importance of offering choice when supporting people with learning disabilities. The resistance to 'doing something different' was felt by all and was passed on to Josh's direct supporters who increased the choices offered to Josh, thus leading to a less comfortable situation for him and increased distress. In the ward round conversations I identified potential exit points at the 'organisational cultural story' level in the loop (we talked in ways which drew attention to the inherent tensions in the various ways in which supporters are told 'what is expected' and the limited operationalisation of the concept of 'meaningful choice'). There also seemed to be exit opportunities at the 'feeling' level of the loop by creating a context where the anxiety which *everyone* was feeling could be acknowledged, and at the identity level by allowing for gentle discussion of the 'inadequate practitioner' identity story which can follow from admission and can push towards adherence to actually quite vague conceptualisations of what it is that supporters 'should be doing', perhaps at the expense of really being able to hear Josh's feedback about what works for him.

Josh settled well into the ATU. He appeared to benefit from the routine and structure which the team understood as creating an enabling context for him given his autism. Incidents of distress reduced dramatically and within a few months Josh was no longer taking any anti-psychotic medication. His family were visiting regularly and taking him out for a pleasurable family day out most weekends. He was enjoying regular trips out with staff, enjoying cooking his favourite meals on regular occasions, and had become very popular with most of the ATU team. This, however, led to the establishing of another strange loop which focused on the 'institutional' nature of a service like an ATU (see Figure 11.2).

Professionals responsible for setting up new services in the community were aware that things were going well for Josh and together the ATU and community staff were keen to set up a new service in the community which could continue to meet Josh's needs in the longer term. There was initial engagement with the idea of recreating some aspects of the support he was receiving, and a willingness to create support plans which guided new staff to, for example, offer limited choice, maintain a more sparse physical environment and structured access to his clothes and toiletries, and there was also an ability to see that in this context Josh appeared to feel safe and secure and to therefore be able to engage with others and with his world. However, when these plans created a context within which anxiety was relieved, the practitioners defaulted to discourses about 'choice, homely environments and control' with narrow interpretations of these ideas based on the assumption that there are cross-cultural, generic and universally shared ideas about what would be a real choice, a homely environment or about what control 'everyone' would want. The staff who support people in learning disability services are often acutely aware of some of the awful ways in

Organisational cultural story: Learning disability services have been institutional in the past and this is bad.

Relationship story: We should not restrict people and we should provide homely environments.

Identity story: I will be a better practitioner than people were in the past.

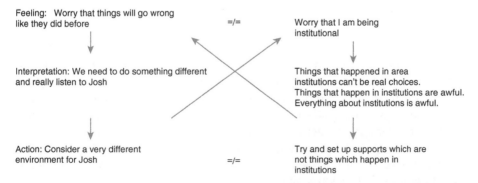

Feeling: Worry that things will go wrong like they did before

=/=

Worry that I am being institutional

Interpretation: We need to do something different and really listen to Josh

Things that happened in area institutions can't be real choices. Things that happen in institutions are awful. Everything about institutions is awful.

Action: Consider a very different environment for Josh

=/=

Try and set up supports which are not things which happen in institutions

Figure 11.2 Institutional approaches to deinstitutionalisation strange loop

which people with learning disabilities services have been treated in the past (see Box 11.4). Strong commitments to never repeating these atrocities can unwittingly give life to narrow interpretations of what people might need. This led to practitioners recommending supports for Josh which were the same as the ones in place before admission. Conversations which deconstructed ideas about 'institutionalisation', 'homeliness', 'choice' and 'control' and allowed a more nuanced and individualised consideration of what Josh may actually have been telling us he needed and wanted allowed for this loop to be exited and a more clear plan communicated with his new staff team which both met Josh's needs and established a foundation for empowering and truly person-centred support. The exit was perhaps at the 'relationship' level as the focus shifted from 'doing what we are told we should do' to 'doing what seems to work for Josh'. The plans allowed for the aspects of his environment and support which were working for Josh to be continued and the bits which were not to be discontinued.

Box 11.4 Find out about the history of services to people with learning disabilities

If you are not aware of the history of learning disability services and of the appalling impact of institutionalisation you may find it helpful to find out more about this. Jenny Webb's chapter 'The Historical Context' in her 2014 book is a great place to start. You may also find it thought provoking (but also potentially very traumatic) to watch 'The Silent Minority' which gives a good insight into what institutions for people with learning disability could be like and may help to promote an understanding of the collective trauma at the history of services which I think is felt by many service users, families and staff. You can access it at: https://www.concordmedia.org.uk/products/the-silent-minority-1167.

Conclusion

Systemic ideas can be very useful in ATU settings. They can, of course, be used in standard ways in individual and family therapeutic sessions. However, they also offer a good framework to both understand the dominant discourses in an ATU setting and also to offer some opportunities to allow for conversations alongside them which ensure that the ATU context is one which can hear and respect the person's views and the meaning of events for them and their family. Thickening of some stories, including stories of diagnosis, can create opportunities for more optimistic futures and can be a part of the 'difference that makes a difference'.

Further questions

➤ What do you see as the pros and cons of seeing problems as being inside a person?

➤ Does it feel OK to use systemic ideas without telling people this is what you are doing?

➤ What other theories and ideas might you be using in your practice without telling people this is what you are doing?

➤ When is it OK to challenge gently and indirectly and when should we challenge ideas more directly?

➤ What other aspects of the contexts and history of ATUs and learning disability services might be influential when a person is admitted to an ATU?

Acknowledgement

With thanks to Celia Heneage for her support in writing this chapter.

References

Bateson, G. (1972). *Steps to an Ecology of Mind*. Chicago, IL: The University of Chicago Press.

Baum, S. & Lynggard, H. (2006). *Intellectual Disabilities: A Systemic Approach*. London: Karnac Books.

Cronen, V. (1994). Coordinated management of meaning: Practical theory for the complexities and contradictions of everyday life. In J. Siegfried (ed.), *The Status of Common Sense in Psychology*, (pp. 183–207). Norwood, OH: Ablex.

Department of Health *Code of Practice - Mental Health Act* (1983) *(First published 15 January 2015, updated 26 March 2015)*. Norwich: The Stationery Office.

Freedman, J. & Combs, G. (1996). *Narrative Therapy: The Social Construction of Preferred Realities*. London: W.W. Norton & Company.

Gehart, D. (2016). *Theory and Treatment Planning in Family Therapy: A Competency-Based Approach*. Boston, MA: Cengage Learning.

Haydon-Laurelut, M. (2015). Disability beyond individualization, psychologisation and medicalization. *Metalogos*, 27, 1–15.

Hayward, M. (2009), Is narrative therapy systemic?, *Context*, October, 13–16.

Holmgren, A. (2004). Saying, doing and making: Teaching CMM theory. *Human Systems: The Journal of Systemic Consultation and Management*, 15, 89–100.

Johnstone, L. (2000). *Users and Abusers of Psychiatry: A Critical Look at Psychiatric Practice,* 2nd edition. London: Routledge.

Mason, B. (1989). *Handing Over: Developing Consistency across Shifts in Residential and Health Settings*. London: Karnac Books (Ltd).

NHS England (2015). *Building the Right Support: A National Plan to Develop Community Services and Close Inpatient Facilities for People with a Learning*

Disability and/or Autism who Display Behaviours that Challenges, including those with a Mental Health Condition. London: NHS England.

NHS England (2017). *Care and Treatment Reviews (CTRs): Policy and Guidance including Policy and Guidance on Care, Education and Treatment Reviews (CETRs) for Children and Young People*. https://www.england.nhs.uk/wp-content/uploads/2017/03/ctr-policy-v2.pdf (accessed 8 January 2019).

Oliver, C. (2004). Reflexive inquiry and the strange loop tool. *Human Systems: The Journal of Systemic Consultation & Management*, 15, 127–140.

Pearce, W.B. (2007). *Making Social Worlds: A Communication Perspective*. Oxford: Blackwell.

Pearce, W.B. (2012). Evolution and transformation: A brief history of CMM and a meditation on what using it does to us. In C. Creede, B. Fisher-Yoshida & P. Gallegos (eds), *The Reflective, Facilitative and Interpretive Practices of the Coordinated Management of Meaning* (p. 1–22). Maryland: Rowman & Littlefield Publishers, Incorporated.

Walther, S. & Fox, H. (2012). Narrative therapy and outsider witness practice: Teachers as a community of acknowledgement. *Educational & Child Psychology*, 29(2), 9–17.

Webb, J. (2014). *A Guide to Psychological Understanding of People with Learning Disabilities: Eight Domains and Three Stories*. Hove: Routledge.

White, M. & Epston, D. (1990). *Narrative Means to Therapeutic Ends*. London: W.W. Norton & Company Ltd.

Wilcox, E., Finlay, W.M. & Edmonds, J. (2006). 'His brain is totally different': An analysis of care-staff explanations of aggressive challenging behaviour and the impact of gendered discourses. *British Journal of Social Psychology*, 45, 197–216.

Wooffitt, R. (1992). *Telling Tales of the Unexpected: The Organization of Factual Discourse*. Hertfordshire: Harvester Wheatsheaf.

Zigmond, T. (2014). *A Clinician's Brief Guide to the Mental Health Act*, 3rd edition. London: RCPsych Publications.

Notes

1   These concepts are, of course, clearly socially constructed but will be used here for brevity. Systemic thinking draws our attention to the importance of language in creating realities and meanings. I've used quotation marks in this chapter on occasion to draw attention to some very strong ideas which nevertheless should not be seen as 'real'; rather, they are constructed through social interactions.

2   The factsheet about learning disabilities produced by BILD gives some very useful information about what people mean when they talk about different severities of learning disabilities: www.bild.org.uk/resources/factsheets.

3   This is not a description of a single piece of real work, but I talk about it as if it is to make it more readable.

12

Guide to a Good Day (G2GD) – A Wellness Recovery Action Plan (WRAP) for People with Learning Disabilities and Their Support Network

Darren Bleek and Lloyd Purdy

Accessible summary

- Wellness Recovery Action Plan (WRAP) is a tool used in mainstream mental health services as a way for people to plan and record actions and habits that support wellness.

- *Guide to a Good Day* (G2GD) has been developed separately from WRAP but does many of the same things for staff teams supporting people with learning disabilities who show behaviours that challenge services.

- G2GD follows a simple traffic light – green, amber, red – structure for increasing the chance of a good day.

- In this chapter we describe how systemic approaches are suited to using G2GD and show G2GD's opportunities for practitioners in a practical, step-by-step way.

Recovery as a movement in mental health circles has arisen from the service user movement in the 1980s and 1990s in the USA and grown to the point where it has been adopted internationally as policy in England (2001/2011), Ireland (2005) and Scotland (2006), New Zealand (1998), the USA (2003), Australia (2003) and Canada (2009) (Roberts & Boardman, 2013).

'Recovery is about building a meaningful and satisfying life, as defined by the person themselves, whether or not there are ongoing or recurring symptoms or problems … a person can recover their life, without necessarily "recovering from" their illness.' (Shepherd et al., 2008) In this sense there are parallels for people living with learning disabilities who seek a fulfilling life despite the presence of disabilities, and recovery model ideas and tools may be of interest to learning disabilities practitioners.

Shepherd et al. (2008) go on to list the principles of recovery. These include a recognition that sometimes the solutions that mental health services and society offer can be part of the problem and so the recovery movement seeks to move away from pathology and deficit towards hope, strengths, and quality of life as defined by the person themselves. It emphasises self-management as a process of discovery of what works for each person in their unique experience. It recognises that recovery is not possible in isolation and that involvement of social networks and social inclusion in society at large forms an important context for supporting well-being. Recovery is co-created where clinicians and helpers are invited to be coaches or partners in this process of discovery rather than experts on top. The language used, the stories told and the meanings that are constructed are central to the recovery process – how these are documented and shared and who owns them can make all the difference to hope and the action taken leading to positive change.

Systemic practitioners will read this description of the recovery movement and should instantly recognise multiple tenets of systemic social constructionist approaches (Anderson & Goolishian, 1988; Hoffman, 2002) and narrative therapy in particular (Freedman & Combs, 1996). Central to narrative therapy is the power of language, stories and therapeutic documents in effecting change (Freedman & Combs, 1996). From this perspective, the *Wellness Recovery Action Plan (WRAP)* could be seen as an example of a therapeutic document that is increasingly used in recovery-oriented mental health services.

At the same time, clinicians working with adults with learning disabilities will recognise echoes of concepts such as the social construction of disability (Goodley, 2011) and a rights-based model of disability that has underpinned parallel initiatives in the past 20 years of deinstitutionalisation, community-based care, inclusion, and government policy in the UK such *as Valuing People* (2001) and *Valuing People Now* (2009). These attitudes and approaches have correspondingly shown up in person-centred support documents such as *Person-Centred Plans* (Sanderson et al., 1997) which value similar principles of empowerment, enablement and social inclusion. As learning disabilities services have operated largely in isolation from mainstream mental health services, the adaptation of tools such as WRAP for people with learning disabilities and additional mental health difficulties or challenging behaviour has not to our knowledge been common practice. In keeping with the parallel development of mental health and learning disabilities services in the UK, we share in this chapter a tool called *Guide to a Good Day (G2GD)* for use in supporting staff teams who present in crisis along with an adult with learning disabilities and behaviour described as challenging. We will show how G2GD is similar to WRAP despite being developed completely independently, and we will also show how it may be a useful tool for practitioners who are interested in working systemically with learning disabilities.

Stories of WRAP – recovery and G2GD in South Devon

G2GD was developed by Zoe Anderson over a number of years from 2005 while the authors were working in a newly formed Community Learning Disabilities Service in South and West Devon. At the time, new perspectives were being created on how to engage in a meaningful way with people with learning disabilities who lived in our community and presented behaviours that challenged, and were at risk of hospitalisation or breakdown in their community support. As the service started to develop, the theme emerged that while the person who had learning disabilities gained access to the service, it was the person's system that we were working with. Zoe Anderson and others in the team were dissatisfied with previous behavioural service work where a more expert approach would result in lengthy reports being written and subsequently filed with apparently frequent re-referral rates. In order to increase treatment sustainability 'what we needed to do was to give our skills away and adopt a less of a protectionist approach hiding behind our long words and clever essays' (Anderson, 2017). When Char Smith, a local speech and language therapist with an interest in solution-focused approaches, joined the team she was already writing communication profiles in an accessible, strengths-oriented way. Other members of the team included the authors (a psychiatrist with additional training in systemic family therapy and a nurse with additional cognitive behavioural therapy (CBT) training) as well as an occupational therapist. Over time these strands were drawn together both philosophically and functionally and *Guide to a Good Day* (G2GD) was developed: a multidisciplinary, multi-functional tool which at its very heart hears the voice of the person and their support network in informing what is needed to co-create the conditions for a 'Good Day'; a tool where the process of arriving at what defines a 'Good Day' for that person and the steps needed to achieve or maintain it are just as important as the final product; a tool that over time has been used with success locally in avoiding hospitalisation and supporting clients to increase good days and help staff teams to support in more positive ways surrounding moments of difficulty.

Unknown to Zoe Anderson and her team, in 1997 Mary Ellen Copeland had published *Wellness Recovery Action Plan* (WRAP). This shifted the position of the professional as the expert, and very much 'allowed' the voice of the person with the lived experience to be heard and define their own experience of mental un-wellness and what helps them. WRAP offered people with this lived experience a tool to state what helped them to maintain their wellbeing and what others might do to support them when things were not so good.

See Information Box 12.1 for more recovery-oriented resources.

Box 12.1 Recovery oriented resources

Recovery Devon
　A gateway to recovery-based support, research and guidance: https://recovery-devon.co.uk

Mary Ellen Copeland
　Personal story of the origins of WRAP:
　Part 1: www.youtube.com/watch?v=JOH5fps4Vpo
　Part 2: www.youtube.com/watch?v=G6xMN57K0xU

Pat Deegan
　Personal story of education and living with schizophrenia: www.youtube.com/watch?v=DVlhfuKDjYE

　Recovery lecture four-minute clip: www.youtube.com/watch?v=jhK-7DkWaKE

　Social barriers careers of mental patients: www.youtube.com/watch?v=vmdZo-G1DFE

At some point in 2011 the authors became aware of recovery concepts and WRAP as a personal recovery tool. The parallels with concepts long held in learning disabilities work were immediately apparent and led to the recognition of synchronistic similarities and differences between our own G2GD and WRAP.

What does *Guide to a Good Day* look like?

G2GD is a deceptively simple tool that uses familiar red/amber/green traffic light colours to support people with learning disabilities and their support network to identify differing states that may require different interactions to increase the chance of a 'Good Day' for all involved.

Simply put, green equals what you may look like when you are well, amber when things are becoming a little more difficult and red when you are in crisis. There is a final section which documents any routines or specific activities which help contribute towards a good day. The design is fun and colourful. The content is practically oriented.

The questions used to generate the descriptions are generally solution-focused, emphasise behaviour as a communication, and draw attention to the context or interactions that increase the chance of a 'Good Day' (but do not guarantee this). It is written in the everyday language that the person with learning disabilities or their support network uses. It is created through a process of interviewing the person's network – those people who make the most sense of the world for the person and whose skills are the ones that need to be refined and developed to create change for the referred person. G2GD works best when the interviewer has identified the small group of people who are invested in and motivated to create change for the person (Anderson, 2017). The content may be influenced by professional opinion but this is done in a collaborative manner with the staff group – sharing skills and experience in an engaging manner as part of the interviewing process or in subsequent support staff training or meetings. The initial G2GD is written by the professional team but it is handed over to the network to take ownership of future updates and revisions.

G2GD sections and headings (see appendix at the end of this chapter for detailed example):

GREEN: (these headings and the text of the document are presented in green)

How I communicate 'like'/'OK'/'happy'

Things I like

Things you need to think about to help me feel OK:

Environment or room:

My understanding:

How I communicate:

How I make choices:

How I initiate/take the lead:

AMBER: (these headings and the text of the document are presented in amber)

Things to avoid:

Things I dislike

How I communicate I am beginning to feel 'dislike'/'anxious'/'bored' or 'finish'

It helps me if you:

RED: (these headings and the text of the document are presented in red)

How I communicate I am feeling 'very anxious'/'angry'

It helps me if you:

ROUTINES: (these headings and the text of the document are presented in green)

Beginnings and endings of my day:

Morning

Afternoon

Evening

Activities: Things you need to think about to help me take part

The people that helped me to produce this document were: (text of this section usually in black)

In contrast if you were to follow the chapter headers for a WRAP in Mary Ellen Copeland's 1997 publication they would be:

➤ Develop a Wellness Toolbox

➤ Daily Maintenance Plan

➤ Triggers

➤ Early Warning Signs (Wake Up Calls)

➤ When things are breaking down

➤ Crisis Planning

➤ Post Crisis Plan

Given that these two documents occurred without knowledge of each other, it is interesting that they seem to share a common approach and a shared understanding of what it is useful to write down.

Stepwise process for creating G2GD and links to systemic practice

How one goes about creating a G2GD, however, is more important than the information under each heading or question, and this is where opportunities for systemic application arise. Table 12.1 sets out the sequence of practical steps taken in developing a G2GD and links these to common systemic practices.

Table 12.1   The sequence of practical steps taken in developing a G2GD and the links to systemic practices

Practical Steps	Systemic Practice
Guide to a Good Day Questions/template is left with relevant members of the support network to review before involvement of professionals.	This warms the context and invites the network to start becoming curious about the questions, to reflect, to engage in inner and outer dialogue.
A member of the professional team goes through the G2GD questions in person with members of the support network. This can be done with individuals or with groups of the support network. If the person with learning disabilities is able to participate in contributing directly to the G2GD then they are consulted as well.	The manner in which these interviews are conducted is crucial – the stance is 'journalistic', maintaining a tension between curiosity, neutrality and therapeutic intent. The questions themselves are inherently solution-focused and seek to draw out narratives of what supports and contributes to a 'Good Day' – this stands in contrast to dominant narratives of defeat and 'offensive' behaviour and invites new meanings.
Various members of a multidisciplinary team concurrently perform their own assessments or direct observations of the system and interactions, e.g. speech and language; occupational therapy; psychiatry; psychology.	Interviews with groups of the support network are preferred as this allows the observation of difference and the sharing of multiple perspectives.
	Previously disempowered members of the social network are given voice – whether family members, paid carers, or the person living with learning disabilities. Wherever possible, and with the assistance of communication experts such as speech and language therapists if needed, the person with learning disabilities is consulted to contribute towards the guide. This approach allows an experience-near description of the problems encountered, values, aspirations, and what helps to be included in the solutions.
	Through this process of multiple interviews and exploration of the situation – the sharing of perspectives, empowerment of previously disempowered elements of the network, and solution-focused enquiry, change is often

Table 12.1 *Continued*

Practical Steps	Systemic Practice
	anecdotally noticed before the tool is fully completed, supporting the systemic notion that the 'assessment is the intervention' and correlates can be made with Karl Tomm's 'interventive interviewing' (Tomm, 1987a, 1987b, 1988).
	Systemic practice values multiple perspectives and this includes the voices and expertise of professionals whilst being mindful that these voices don't overpower those of the person and their support network. The perspectives of the multidisciplinary team are included in the final G2GD document in a supportive and solution-focused manner and tied in with additional therapeutic interventions outside of the guide.
The various responses to the G2GD questions are collated into a unified final draft version which includes the perspectives of multidisciplinary assessments. All statements in the guide are written in the first person, as if they are said by the identified person with learning disabilities.	A member of the professional team has initial editorial control over drafting the document. This stands in direct contrast to the authorship of a WRAP in mainstream mental health services where the document is written by the person with mental health problems. In learning disabilities circles, others step in to this role to assist where an individual is not fully capable – allowing the person to 'borrow' the words and executive function offered by professionals and others in their support network to complete this task. Wherever possible, however, the words and perspective of the person living with learning disabilities should be privileged.
	Whilst the professional collating the documents cannot escape their own inherent biases, maintaining an element of self-reflexivity regarding this as well as inviting review from other members of the professional team and the support network are important safeguards to have in place.
	The draft is written with therapeutic intent and maintains the stance of producing a solution-focused document with an emphasis on the various contexts that support a 'Good Day' – communication, routines, interactions, relationships, factors in the physical environment. This supports a reframe that emphasises a social construction of disability and distressed behaviour and shifts negative attributions in the system. It pays attention to the power of

Table 12.1 *Continued*

Practical Steps	Systemic Practice
	language – using as much of the words and descriptions offered by the person and their support network as possible.
The final version of the G2GD is taken back to the support network and presented in a group context for implementation – this is often usefully framed as a training event for paid carers but offers an opportunity for further dialogue about its contents (and possible revision).	The G2GD is a living document. It requires those most intimately involved with its contents to take ownership and responsibility for review and revision in the future. This is only possible if it is understood and if those involved feel able to influence its contents – even at a final stage.
Further training events might flow from this if there are specific topics where this is agreed to be useful e.g. carers may wish to be educated further on autism; or there may be specific communication techniques or approaches that could benefit from further training or therapeutic intervention.	The G2GD is the centrepiece of the multidisciplinary team's work with an individual and their support network. It often creates the reason and relevance for engagement in further therapeutic interventions.
Working with hierarchy to mobilise resources and support needed for change.	From a structural perspective it is important to recognise and value hierarchy in the functioning of a system. Many people with learning disabilities live in a nested eco-system of hierarchy that includes family members, managers and owners of care homes or support organisations, and local social care managers and commissioners of support services.
	Pursuing a solution-focused support plan will often require changes to resourcing or ways of working that require the endorsement of those in authority or with power and control at various levels of the wider care system. Incorporating the G2GD into formal care plans; gaining the support and cooperation of managers of private providers; and ensuring the plans are funded and commissioned by health and social care teams is an important clinical advocacy task that requires attention.
Helping the support network to own the document and its review.	This is a thread which is woven throughout the creation of a G2GD. From the beginning it is important to ensure members feel they are making a meaningful contribution and the document belongs to them.
	At the initial implementation it is helpful to have an identified person in the support network who is made responsible for keeping the G2GD up to date – this could be a key worker in a paid support network or a close family member in the family home setting.

Concluding thoughts

It should be apparent to the reader that the G2GD does not ask any ground-breaking questions of the person or their network, nor does it necessarily readily identify with any specific model of intervention. What we have sought to do here is share this new tool through the lens of systemic theory and practice for anyone interested in ways of applying this to their work with people with learning disabilities. We have also sought to demonstrate the parallels between G2GD and WRAP – both of which have similar orientations towards empowerment of service users in relation to help and the social construction of disability or well-being. While WRAP is primarily focused on the individual and their self-management in the socio-political context of living with mental health challenges, G2GD chooses to focus attention on the support network surrounding a person living with learning disabilities who shows distressed or challenging behaviour. It does this by providing a simple structure and focal point for potentially complex interventions.

Box 12.2 Reflective questions on using a guide to a good day

- In our team most of the interviews to gather information for the G2GD are conducted by support workers rather than professionally qualified systemic therapists. If you were to do the same, what qualities would you encourage in the interviewer or what systemic techniques might it be helpful to teach the interviewer if you were supervising their work?

- Reviewing the process for creating a G2GD, can you identify what levels or parts of the system surrounding a person with learning disabilities may need to be engaged with?

- If you were to use the G2GD in your own practice, who might you need to recruit as allies or collaborators to complete the tool from start to finish?

- How might you see the language of a 'good day' being more helpful than the language of a 'good life' or a 'good person'?

- The G2GD values multiple perspectives; how would you include the views of professionals while still privileging the voice and experience of the person with learning disabilities and their support network who know them best and help them to make sense of the world?

Appendix: Sample Guide to a Good Day

This is a composite example of a G2GD for a fictitious person drawn from the work and experience of the authors.

GREEN:

How I communicate 'like'/'OK'/'happy'

I will give you a thumbs up or a smile/I will laugh and perhaps tell a joke/ point to show something I want to talk to you about/I will smile (showing my teeth)

Make happy noises

Things I like

I like going to the park and especially on the swings or slides

Birds and wildlife programmes

Dogs and other animals

Things you need to think about to help me feel OK

I like going to the beach

Bubble tubes in my sensory room

Environment or room:

If there are a few people around, it helps if only one person takes the lead in communicating with me

I like a lot of personal space

My understanding:

I don't use much speech – I need people to help me to show that I am interested as I won't always tell you

Using objects to support what you are saying can also help me to understand what you are saying. I will touch an object to say that I want it, or push it away to say that I don't

How I communicate:

I can sometimes use familiar words or phrases to tell you what I want, e.g. eggs and soldiers

I will touch something or use my eyes to direct towards something and choose something

How I make choices:

I won't initiate any activities

I need others to ask me whether I need anything or want to do anything

I will need full prompting with most activities

I use vocalisations to get your attention and show you something or tell you that something is distressing me

AMBER:

Things to avoid

Being rushed at meals – I am a slow eater and need plenty of prompting

Giving me too many options. I can choose between two things if the options are simple and clear

Don't let me know about things that are going to happen until you know all the details – I will worry about arrangements

People who I think make changes in my life (e.g. doctors, social workers) can make me anxious. Make their meetings feel positive by arranging to go out for a drink and cake afterwards

Things I dislike

I don't like swimming

Being too hot

How I communicate I am beginning to feel 'dislike'/'anxious'/'bored' or 'finish'

I will start slapping my thighs

I will move in a jerky way – mainly head

It helps me if you:

Stay with me and give me 1:1 time to help me take part in an activity

Give instructions that are direct and clear and in context

Use short sentences and use objects to help when you talk to me

RED:

How I communicate I am feeling 'very anxious'/'angry'

I will talk more and will repeat what others say

I bang or hit walls

I will repeat requests for things or specific people

I can remain in a distressed state for up to two hours

It helps me if you:

Stay calm and confident

Use less speech as I tend not to follow what you're saying

Keep communication to a minimum

Involve me in solving the problem

Following an incident I must be allowed to apologise. Everyone must say 'Yeah okay, I accept your apology'

ROUTINES:

Beginnings and endings of my day:

Morning:

Cup of tea

Listen to music

Bath and then get dressed

Afternoon:

I like to 'chill out'/have time on my own

Evening:

I like to cook tea

I have my bath at about 8.30/8.45pm

I go to bed around 9.00pm and watch DVDs

Activities: Things you need to think about to help me take part

Have everything ready before you offer me the activity

Tell me about any changes to my routine using speech. Any planned changes or when new routine are introduced should be in small steps, e.g. show me photographs of where I'm going beforehand

You may need to hold my hand or place your hand over mine

The people that helped me to produce this document were:

Parents

Support team

Day services

References

Anderson, H. & Goolishian, H. (1988). Human systems as linguistic systems: Preliminary and evolving ideas about the implications for clinical theory. *Family Process*, 27(4), 371–393.

Anderson, Z. (2017). Personal communication.

Copeland, ME (1997, revised 2000). Wellness Recovery Action Plan. Peach Press, USA.

Department of Health (2001). *Valuing People: A New Strategy for Learning Disability for the 21st Century*. London: Department of Health.

Department of Health (2009). *Valuing People Now: a new three-year strategy for people with learning disabilities – 'making it happen for everyone'*. https://webarchive.nationalarchives.gov.uk/20130105064234/http://www.dh.gov.uk/prod_consum_dh/groups/dh_digitalassets/documents/digitalasset/dh_093375.pdf (accessed 25 February 2019).

Freedman, J. & Combs, G. (1996). *Narrative Therapy – The Social Construction of Preferred Realities*. New York: W.W. Norton & Company Inc.

Goodley, D. (2011). *Disability Studies – An Interdisciplinary Introduction*. London: Sage Publications Ltd.

Hoffman, L. (2002). *Family Therapy – An Intimate History*. New York: W.W. Norton & Company Inc.

Roberts, G. & Boardman, J. (2013). Understanding 'recovery'. *Advances in Psychiatric Treatment*, 19, 400–409.

Sanderson, H., Kennedy, J., Ritchie, P. & Goodwin, G. (1997). *People, Plans and Possibilities: Exploring Person-Centred Planning*. Edinburgh: SHS Trust.

Shepherd, G., Boardman, J. & Slade, M. (2008). *Making Recovery a Reality*. Sainsbury Centre for Mental Health. https://www.meridenfamilyprogramme.com/download/recovery/tools-for-recovery/Making_recovery_a_reality_policy_paper.pdf (accessed 25 February 2019).

Tomm, K. (1987a). Interventive interviewing: Part I. Strategizing as a fourth guideline for the therapist. *Family Process*, 26, 3–13.

Tomm, K. (1987b). Interventive interviewing: Part II. Reflexive questioning as a means to enable self-healing. *Family Process*, 26, 153–183.

Tomm, K. (1988). Interventive interviewing: Part III. Intending to ask lineal, circular, reflexive or strategic questions? *Family Process*, 27, 1–15.

13

When Someone Dies: Practices of Witnessing and Re-membering

Henrik Lynggaard and Bethan Ramsey

Accessible summary

- When someone dies it can be useful for people to get together to have what is called a re-membering conversation.

- This kind of conversation can help us to talk about important relationships in our lives.

- It is important to make careful preparations for such conversations.

- Letters can be a good way to catch, name and give ideas and learnings back to people who have told their stories.

- It is very important to adapt our ways of working to the people we meet rather than trying to adapt people to what we do.

'I hope Mary doesn't die on my shift,' Sally said.

Mark looked relieved. 'I've been thinking exactly the same.'

Sandra agreed. 'It's really time that Mary went in to hospital.'

Sally, Mark and Sandra (not their real names) were support workers in a community home for five residents with learning disabilities, one of whom, Mary, had advanced dementia and was not expected to live long. Their comments were made in one of the regular meetings about Mary's support. Although Sally, Mark and Sandra expressed reservations about their ability to care for someone dying at home, other professionals involved with Mary, including the 24-hour palliative care service, were impressed by the skilled care offered to her. Likewise, Mary's family were keen she should spend the remaining period of her life in the place that had been her home for the past 20 years. They knew that there was no other setting where she would be offered anything approaching the level of individualised care she was currently receiving. They said that a move to a strange or unfamiliar place, with staff who did not know anything about Mary, her life and her preferences, was likely to lead to a rapid deterioration in her quality of life. However, as can be seen, Sally, Mark and Sandra had felt it important to speak of her unease of death occurring on their shift. As the conversation progressed, they spoke of their worry that they would be blamed or criticised for not acting in the right way when offering end-of-life care to Mary and expressed a wish that her death should take place elsewhere.

Shifting attitudes to death and dying in Western societies, from the Middle Ages to modern times, have been studied by many historians. In a seminal work by Ariès (1974), some key developments over the last century are set out: death has progressively become associated with shame and failure; dying 'out of sight' in a hospital is increasingly common and associated with a failure of medicine rather than seen as a normal occurrence; and death is being treated as an illness from which many people, especially children, are shielded. In the context of learning disabilities services, several studies have suggested that support workers are unprepared for the challenges of end-of-life care and are, in Todd's words, 'taken by surprise by its demands, but willing to overcome these to care for people with intellectual disabilities at the end of their lives' (Todd, 2013, p. 216). That Sally, Mark and Sandra's concerns are in no way uncommon can be read from the title that Brown and his colleagues gave to their study 'Please don't let it happen on my shift!' (Brown et al., 2003). The worries of staff are also magnified and fuelled by numerous examples encountered in contemporary public services and amplified in the media when deaths, even expected ones, are treated as a serious incident, triggering investigations and critical scrutiny. Moreover, in this culture of blame, staff's reactions to the death of a person they may have known or cared for intimately for years are minimised or relegated to the sidelines (Ryan et al., 2011).

In this chapter, we introduce some concepts and practices derived from systemic and narrative theories that in our experience can open up conversational possibilities that might not otherwise have existed. We make detailed reference to three examples from our practice as clinical psychologists working in a multidisciplinary community team. In two of these examples feedback affirmed the usefulness of our approach, and in the final example we describe how our assumptions and strong attachment to our method afforded sobering learning.

Re-membering conversations

Michael White (2007) introduced the concept of 're-membering' into narrative therapeutic practices and conversations. Narrative therapy centres people as the experts in their own lives. It views problems as separate from people and assumes that people have many abilities, competencies and beliefs that will assist them to reduce the influence of the problems in their lives (see Morgan, 2000 for an easy-read introduction to narrative therapy). The concept of re-membering refers to how people we are associated with in the course of our lives can be considered as being members of our 'club' of life. Some of the people we will have chosen to be part of our lives; with others we will have had little choice over their inclusion. Morgan (2000) writes:

> When people are faced with a problem, they often experience isolation and disconnection from important relationships. The dominant problem story may be successful in minimising or making invisible certain partnerships or histories in the person's life. Re-membering conversations are intended to redress this […] these conversations provide a direct contrast to many current cultural practices that encourage individualisation and disconnection of people from one another (pp. 77–78).

In our experience there can be a tendency in health and social care services to undervalue relationships and to overvalue procedures and protocols, resulting in staff feeling demoralised and isolated in their work. The practice of re-membering conversations seeks to evoke skills and knowledge that have been co-generated in the significant relationships of a person's life. As Fredman (1997) has emphasised, it is a process that weaves both backwards and forwards 'involv[ing] re-membering of the past into the present so that a context can be created from which to act towards the future' (p. 92). In the next section, using a referral from a residential staff team, we illustrate aspects of our practice inspired by re-membering practices, and some of the questions that we have borrowed or adapted from Fredman (1997) and White (2007). In our account of the first example, we spend some time explaining how we usually respond to new referrals and how we create a context for opening space for dialogue.

Lillian

The referral

Tim, the manager of a small group home, similar in many ways to the one described in the opening paragraph, approached the multidisciplinary learning disabilities team where we are employed as clinical psychologists. Tim explained that Lillian had died four weeks previously after a year-long illness, at the age of 67. Lillian had lived at the home for 10 years and was liked by fellow residents and staff. She had been diagnosed with an aggressive form of cancer that had not responded to treatment. Apart from a brief period in hospital she had remained in her home until she passed away. Tim went on to explain that making arrangements for Lilian's funeral and responding to the reactions and needs of the other residents, in addition to an investigation conducted by the local social service department, had left the staff little time to come together to reflect on Lillian's life and death. Tim asked if we would meet with him and his team to facilitate such a conversation.

Relationship to help questions

When, as systemic and narrative informed practitioners, we receive a request for work, especially when a person is making a referral in respect of someone else (e.g. here a manager on behalf of the team), we find it important to explore the question: Who wants what for whom? For example, if a referral is made for anger management by Jeff's key worker, we do not assume that Jeff shares these concerns or would describe them in the same terms. This is where the 'relationship to help' questions developed by Reder and Fredman (1996) can prove very useful. So in an initial conversation with Tim we asked:

➤ Whose idea was it to ask for the session?

➤ What do other staff think about this?

➤ What do you think the staff would like to get out of the session?

➤ Will staff have a choice in whether they attend?

➤ Have you done anything like this before?

Tim explained that the idea to ask for a facilitator to lead a discussion had arisen in a staff meeting and had met with general agreement. He added that there was no obligation for staff to attend. On the basis of what

Tim told us about how the request had come about, we went ahead and arranged an hour-and-a-half-long meeting with the team. Had we heard that staff had not been consulted, or had expressed reservations about the referral, we would have wanted more conversations to take place before agreeing on the best way in which we could be useful to Tim and his colleagues.

Intentions guiding our approach and questions

In the practices that we describe in this chapter, it is not our intention to act out of a normative idea of how people should react when someone close to them dies. Rather, we start the conversation with questions that evoke the person who has passed away. In this we are informed by White's (1988) metaphor of saying 'Hello again', a conversational move counteracting prevailing cultural notions or requirements of 'moving on' and 'achieving closure'. Secondly, our questions seek to bring forth stories that honour the meaningful relationships which staff have built with the person. Thirdly, our questions are informed by a two-way understanding of lives and relationships; that is, we enquire not only about what staff have contributed to the person's life, but also what the person has contributed to staff members' lives, and what difference this might make to their work with other people.

Establishing a context for talking together

When we meet with groups of people we arrange chairs in a circle so everyone can see and hear each other. After introductions, we ask about people's understanding of why we are meeting. We explain how we work, namely that one of us will facilitate the conversation, while the other person takes some notes so we can remember what we have talked about and capture people's ideas and return these in a letter. This letter also serves as a way of connecting staff who were not able to be present. We further explain that we work as a team and will share some of our thinking in a conversation between us that the staff can listen to. This is called the reflecting team method (Andersen, 1992). We also ask about significant, but absent, staff members. We initiate a discussion about what we need to agree on so that people feel comfortable and respected. For further ideas on how to open space for systemically informed conversations such as this, see Fredman et al. (2010). Below is an outline of the questions that guided us in our discussion with Lillian's staff team.

Box 13.1 Framework for conversation with staff team following request for opportunity to talk about resident who died

1. We did not know Lillian, but we wonder...

    If Lillian was with us today, what do you think she would like us to know about her?

    What words would you use to describe Lillian and the kind of a person she was?

    What do you think Lillian's family/friends would add to these descriptions?

2. When you think about Lillian, what are some of things/memories/stories that come to mind?

3. What are some of the things you are most pleased about in the support you and your colleagues gave to Lillian and/or her family?

4. What do you think *you* have contributed to Lillian and her family's life?

5. In what ways has your life been affected as a result of knowing and working with Lillian?

6. What do you think it would mean to Lillian and/or her family to know that we have had this conversation today?

7. What has it been like having this conversation today? And what difference might it make to your work with other people?

Feedback

We finished the meeting with the staff team by asking for their thoughts about it. Several people said that sharing memories and stories about Lillian's life had made it seem as if she was physically present in the room. Many said that they had appreciated being invited to think about how their lives had been influenced by knowing Lillian. Staff members also spoke at their relief of being invited to talk about things that had gone well in their interactions with Lillian, commenting that it had felt like a breath of fresh air in a climate of blame. Particularly noteworthy was the fact that some people said that the conversation had helped them reconnect with the reasons they had chosen to work with people with learning disabilities in the first place.

Peter

Peter, a 24-year-old man with severe learning disabilities, was living in a respite unit while building work was carried out on his flat. Peter was well known to the staff in the respite home, having used local services for most of his life. One morning Peter was found unconscious on the floor in his room. Only 10 minutes earlier a staff member had greeted Peter in the corridor while he was on his way to use the toilet. Peter had returned the staff member's greeting in his usual cheerful manner, and then returned to his room. Peter was pronounced dead by the ambulance staff and doctor who arrived quickly after they were called. Everybody at the home was in shock. There had been nothing in Peter's behaviour or demeanour in the preceding weeks to indicate that he was unwell. His health had been good for many years. The results of an autopsy and other investigations eventually confirmed that Peter had died from an inherited and rare heart condition known as 'sudden arrhythmic death syndrome'. Several of the staff who had been on shift in the night and on the morning when Peter died were especially affected, asking themselves frequently if there was something they had failed to notice or do, or if their efforts at resuscitation while waiting for the ambulance had not been of a good enough standard. In conversations with their manager, Emma, staff said that they had never before seen a dead person and certainly not someone as young at Peter. In discussion with Emma, the staff team made a request to talk and think more about this startling event.

On receiving this request from the team at the respite unit, we were guided by the approach we have outlined in the first example which included asking questions about who in the team had asked for the meeting, what other staff members thought about this request, and what people might want from our conversation and involvement. In the meeting with seven members of the staff team, we again began by creating a joint context for talking together and then made use of the questions above, but being careful to expand on some or modify others by paying close attention to how the questions touched people. Below we have copied extracts from the letter we sent to the team afterwards. In our writing of these letters we have been influenced by Fox (2003) and Newman (2008) and like those practitioners we seek to extract key themes from the conversation, to capture resonant phrases and, like Newman puts it so well, to 'rescue the said from the saying of it' (p. 24).

Box 13.2 Extracts from a letter recording a reflective staff discussion following a sudden death

'Being part of a play that wasn't rehearsed'

The nature of Peter's death was so sudden and unforeseen, and someone spoke of 'being part of a play that wasn't rehearsed'. You told us of the shock and disbelief that many of you experienced in the time after Peter's death. In spite of this, you went on to talk of how each person found their role, their part in what unfolded. We noticed how, without a script, you emerged more connected and bonded as a team, at each turn acting with humanity and care.

▶

No time to pause

You told us how, in a busy service like X, even such a big loss does not afford time for pause. Many of you spoke of being pleased with how 'the team pulled together' and 'carried on professionally'. We heard that it was difficult to work, at times scary, but that people were compassionate towards one another. Someone spoke of 'being inspired by the level of support' they saw.

Supporting others as you supported Peter

You told us that you feel Peter has left something of a legacy, which you wished to continue to honour. You told us that he was very assertive about getting his needs met, and that you would like to continue to support others as you supported Peter. We heard much about what this support would look like:

- Having an open-door policy to service users, being a client-led environment.
- Listening carefully to people's voices and responding quickly.
- Keeping consistency, as Peter appreciated consistency in his support.
- Encouraging clients to be expressive.
- Finding ways to connect with people, even where language is limited, using touch and gesture.

We heard that Peter's infectious way of life continues to live on in many ways.

One of you spoke of how his death at such a young age had inspired you to think that life should be lived to the full.

As we ended our meeting, we wondered whether other teams might have something to learn from your hard-earned experiences? We wondered if you might share it with other colleagues across the district, or whether you would give us permission to talk to others about what we learnt from you, without, of course, disclosing any of your individual details?

Feedback following meeting

The day after the staff had received the letter, we received a call from the manager who thanked us for facilitating the meeting and for the letter we had sent. Emma informed us that the meeting and the letter had been significant to the staff team and that it had had a noticeable impact on the atmosphere in the unit. She said that people had felt dejected, incompetent and burdened by a sense of failure. While not minimising the seriousness of what had happened, Emma explained that the way we had conducted the conversation had enabled staff to reconnect with what was important to them in their work. Emma had noticed that the meeting had highlighted that, far from being paralysed, the staff team had in fact come together and been able to draw on their collective skills and knowledge. She further described that the letter had given a way of connecting the night staff, who had not been able to be present, but who had formed an important connection with Peter. Emma also explained that one member of staff who had been most closely involved when Peter died had sought further support from the organisation's counselling service as the death had powerfully evoked a previous bereavement. It was heartening for us to hear back from Emma a year later, when in another correspondence she wrote that she had continued to reflect on our work together, stating: 'Your support provided such a meaningful space for everyone to explore the different ways they managed this very sad and unexpected event.'

Rosie

The third, and final, example is included as a cautionary note against according a higher priority to our favoured methods and techniques over and above the particularity of the situation, or the people, we are meeting with. Four months after the work that we described in our first example, we were again contacted by Tim. He explained that, in an adjacent home, which was part of the same organisation, Rosie, a 59-year-old resident with a diagnosis of dementia, had recently died after a long illness. Like Lillian and Mary, Rosie had been cared for in her home with the support of many specialist services. We knew of Rosie, as members from our multidisciplinary service had been involved in providing input for some years. We agreed to the request to facilitate a meeting similar in format to the one undertaken in respect of Lillian. However, this time we did not ask our usual relationship to help questions (see above, in Lillian's case), assuming that discussion prior to the referral had taken place within the staff team, and that our re-membering conversation framework would have as good a fit as it had with the sister home. We also shortened the time we gave to setting the context for the discussion. So when starting our conversation with the three members of staff, Grace, Elizabeth and Zana, our first question met with an unexpected response:

Henrik: We have heard of Rosie, but never met her. Could you tell us a bit about the kind of person she was?

Grace: I don't really want to talk about Rosie.

Elizabeth: No, it seems far too late. I don't know why we couldn't have had this meeting when she was still alive.

Grace: Yes, that is right. And I don't want to get all upset again.

Henrik: I'm sorry. I think Bethan and I have come along today carrying some big assumptions with us. Do you mind if we start over again? [Some nodding, that I took as permission to go on] ... I would like to begin by asking each of you what ideas you have about why we are meeting?

Elizabeth: To talk about our feelings about Rosie's death. Yeah, like bereavement counselling, because management think we are not coping.

Zana: Yes, about why we have all been so upset.

Henrik: I think I have a sense of how upsetting it would be if you had been given the idea that Bethan and I were here today to deliver bereavement counselling; that is, to deliver something that you had not asked for, especially if your wish to have opportunities to talk when Rosie was still alive was not heard. Since we are all here today, would it be OK to see if we can come up with a way of talking together that could be useful to you?

By slowing things down, and taking time to coordinate our actions with the expectations of the team, we were able to co-create an agenda about how our discussion could be most useful to the staff members. As our discussion progressed we learnt a lot about Rosie: heard stories about her life and connections with the staff; about the big changes the illness brought about for Rosie and those who knew her; and about the individual and collective knowledges, abilities and resourcefulness the staff drew on and developed in the course of their work. Our capture and return of these knowledges and creative practices in a written format were welcomed. We later heard that, in spite of the awkward start, people had felt valued as their ideas and resources had been emphasised. However, for us, this meeting generated some important lessons that we would like to highlight; namely the importance of treating each new referral as unique, however much it may resemble one we have encountered before. Moreover, we should not assume that others will share our enthusiasm for our favoured methods. For more on this topic, see Chapter 23 on irreverence.

In the final part of this chapter we highlight some of the processes and developments in contemporary practice that can be dulling of our attention and capacity for what Shotter (2015) has referred to as our 'dialogic responsiveness'. Dialogic responsiveness refers to the importance of being able to respond moment by moment to the concerns and expressions of the people we are in conversation with, rather than being overly guided by a preset agenda.

Evolving living practices versus manualised approaches

History is replete with examples of practices that have been successfully developed in response to a particular set of local circumstances, but which over time become elevated or promoted as a standard to be implemented everywhere. Writing in 1966, Tom Main reflected on an experience two decades earlier while he was working in an innovative therapeutic community. The staff team had debated and discussed the aims of their work and reached the conclusion that patients should be enabled to go home at the weekend if they wished. However, some months later Main was surprised to overhear a member of staff trying to persuade a patient to go home, implying that it was good for all patients to go home at weekends. Main comments:

> The officialese of the hospital was still about patients being free to choose about their weekends, but these words were now mere relics of an idea and no longer representative of a living truth. What had originally been a useful idea and a break from thoughtless discipline was itself becoming a new kind of thoughtless discipline. (1966, p. 62).

Main warns of the danger of allowing a body of knowledge to become, in its passage from one person to another, a mere set of never-to-be-questioned beliefs. We witness much the same phenomena in rigid manualised treatment protocols or heavily prescriptive care pathways that Wilson (2017) has advocated be (hu)manualised. As other people have commented, the very notion of a manual readily evokes the booklet that accompanies a piece of machinery, and if it is followed as a bureaucratic procedure there is a risk of treating people as objects. Much so-called evidence-based practice with its pseudo-scientific veneer and the silencing intent of its master word 'evidence' can similarly have the consequence of turning people into objects or assigning problems to people that have a passing resemblance to descriptions in a manual, but little relevance to the singular situation of the person we meet. As Voruz and Wolf have stated, 'the universalisation of the discourse of science forecloses singularity and thus the dignity of the individual' (2007, pp. xvi–xvii). While there is much we can learn from the inspiring examples and work of others, we need to adapt and use such knowledge in a way that has a fit with the local and specific context and the people we meet or work with. This is why, in systemic and narrative approaches, we spend considerable time coordinating with people we meet with.

Conclusion

In this chapter we have introduced practices and methods developed within systemic and narrative therapy. In particular we have drawn on the framework of re-membering conversations in our work with three staff teams where a resident died. We have described how we respond to referrals, how we try to coordinate a context for talking together, and how we used letters to catch, name and give ideas and learnings back. We have also emphasised the importance of receiving and responding to referrals one by one, adapting our approach to the people we meet with rather than trying to adapt people to our ways of working. It has not been our intention to suggest that the practices we have foregrounded are the only ways of responding to the situations described. However, we hope our examples have shown how re-membering practices can connect and link people together around shared purposes and values.

Box 13.3 Reflective questions on conducting conversations using a framework

Are you involved in a situation where you could envisage taking your bearings from the framework outlined in this chapter?

What would be your hopes and intentions in using this framework?

Who is involved, connected or significant in regard to the work?

What would be your first step, and what preparations would you need to make?

Who could join you in the work?

Who would you need to involve or consult in taking the work forward?

How is the situation you are involved with similar and how it is different to the examples given in this chapter?

References

Andersen, T. (1992). Reflections on reflecting with families. In S. McNamee & K. Gergen (eds), *Therapy as Social Construction*, (pp. 54–68). London: Sage.

Ariès, P. (1974). *Western Attitudes Towards Death: From the Middle Ages to the Present.* Baltimore, MD and London: The Johns Hopkins University Press.

Brown, H., Burns, S. & Flynn, M. (2003). 'Please don't let it happen on my shift!': Supporting staff who are caring for people with learning disabilities who are dying. *Tizard Learning Disabilities Review*, 8, 32–41.

Fox, H. (2003). Using therapeutic documents – A review. *International Journal of Narrative Therapy and Community Work*, 4, 26–36.

Fredman, G. (1997). *Death Talk. Conversations with Children and Families*. London: Karnac Books.

Fredman, G., Anderson, E. & Stott, J. (2010). *Being With Older People: A Systemic Approach*. London: Karnac Books.

Main, T. (1966/1990). Knowledge, learning and freedom from thought. *Psychoanalytic Psychotherapy*, 5, 59–74.

Morgan, A. (2000). *What is Narrative Therapy: An Easy-To-Read Introduction*. Adelaide: Dulwich Centre Publications.

Newman, D. (2008). 'Rescuing the said from the saying of it': Living documentation in narrative therapy. *The International Journal of Narrative Therapy and Community Work*, 3, 24–34.

Reder, P. & Fredman, G. (1996). The relationship to help: Interacting beliefs about the treatment process. *Clinical Psychology and Psychiatry*, 1(3), 457–467.

Ryan, K., Guerin, S., Dodd, P. & McEvoy, J. (2011). End-of-life care for people with intellectual disabilities: Paid carer perspectives. *Journal of Applied Research in Intellectual Disabilities* 24, 199–207.

Shotter, J. (2015). On being dialogical: An ethics of 'attunement'. *Context*, 137, 8–11.

Todd, S. (2013). 'Being there': The experiences of staff in dealing with matters of dying and death in services for people with intellectual disabilities. *Journal of Applied Research in Intellectual Disabilities*, 26, 215–230.

Voruz, V. & Wolf, B. (2007). *The Later Lacan: An Introduction*. Albany: State University of New York Press.

White, M. (1988). Saying hullo again: The incorporation of the lost relationship in the resolution of grief. *Dulwich Centre Newsletter*. 7–11.

White, M. (2007). *Maps of Narrative Practice*. New York: Norton.

Wilson, J. (2017). *Creativity in Times of Constraint: A Practitioner's Companion in Mental Health and Social Care*. London: Karnac.

14

Systemic Ideas in the Context of Supervision and Reflective Practice

Victoria Jones

Accessible summary

- Supervision is a relationship that happens to help people learn and make sure they do their job well.

- Supervision is about support and making sure that people are good enough at their job.

- Systemic supervision thinks about how people do relationships and communication.

- Relational reflection asks us to think about how other people see things and not just how we see things.

O wad some Pow'r the giftie gie us
To see oursels as others see us!
It wad frae monie a blunder free us
An' foolish notion:
What airs in dress an' gait wad lea'e us,
An' ev'n Devotion!
Oh would some Divine Power give us the small gift
To be able to see ourselves as others see us!
It would save us from many a blunder
And foolish thought:
We would change the way we look and pose
And even what we spend time caring about!

Robert Burns, 1786

What is it that makes supervision systemic?

Flaskas (2014) identified 'three Rs' of learning about systemic thinking and techniques: reflection, recursivity and reflexivity. The majority of training programmes for professions that support people take place in the frame of these three concepts (Dallos & Stedmon, 2009). However, many tend to put most of their emphasis on reflective practice, sometimes using it to encompass all three concepts.

There is a wide range of models of reflection, which vary according to the extent to which there is a focus on feelings; experiences; personal values and beliefs; evidence; policies; politics; feedback; learning; and practice. For example, Somerville and Keeling (2004) focus on reflection as a personal process. They suggest that the opportunity for the creation of alternative actions offered by reflective practice is a critical aspect that avoids it becoming an introverted 'navel gazing' activity. Reflection can be considered a process that enables a practitioner to balance both experience and evidence in the pursuit of a best fit for a given situation. Whilst Tate and Sills (2004) see it as using personal and theoretical ways of knowing to explore being in an experience in order to learn from it.

Dallos and Stedmon (2009) suggest that reflection occurs *in* action (when we give in-the-moment attention to what we are doing and why we are doing it), whilst recursivity occurs *on* action (after-the-event consideration of the myriad factors influencing both our actions and our in-the-moment reflections).

We learn through the recursiveness of knowledge, practice, and our use of self what we know and what we think we know (Flaskas, 2014). Reflexivity requires that we account for our own position (i.e. the things that influence us and the way that we mentally approach something or someone) and the effect of our own position in all our reflective processes. It 'lies at the heart of the development of independent thinking about practice theory, and the development of integrative practice which sees practitioners in constant relationship to the knowledge they use and to their own use of self, in the interests of their clients' (Flaskas, 2014, p. 293).

Whilst the Association for Family Therapy (Association for Family Therapy and Systemic Practice in the United Kingdom, 2009) requires its registered supervisors to be able to demonstrate a range of abilities across four domains: practice, theory, personal development and ethics, there are few aspects of its criteria that are specifically identifiable as systemic. Indeed, there are arguably only two items that are not generalisable to any modality of supervision and specifically refer to systemic concepts: one is in the application of relevant systemic theory, and the second criterion relates to the supervisor's ability to:

> Recognise, understand and use patterns from within own significant relationship systems and contexts that may be a constraint or opportunity in clinical practice and supervision.

> (4.3b, p. 5)

Thus, any efficient and effective supervisor who draws on systemic theories whilst also working reflexively with their own relational and contextual knowledge could be said to be offering systemic supervision. But what might that look like?

Approaches to systemic theories in supervision

Most recently, AFT (Association for Family Therapy and Systemic Practice in the United Kingdom, 2016) described supervision as 'a collaborative, reflective and reflexive process, taking place within the context of a working relationship', and added that a key function of supervision is the 'facilitation of a culture of self and relational reflexivity to enhance clinical and professional practice'. However, Cullen (2017, p. 152) cites an earlier AFT (2011) document that defines supervision as a 'formal process of professional support and learning which enables individuals to develop knowledge and with confidence, assume responsibility for their own practice and enhance consumer protection and safety of care'.

These are arguably complementary but somewhat different definitions, with the first focusing on a mutual process to enhance practice and the latter stressing protection of the public and good practice through a process of learning and guidance. There is some commonality here with the ideas of Shaw (2013) who considered the balance between mentoring and monitoring as the art and challenge of systemic supervision. She suggested that these concepts enabled a systemic model that highlighted the range of stakeholders with a vested interest in good practice outcomes and clinical governance – employers, commissioners, taxpayers, therapists, supervisors and, of course, clients. She emphasised the need for supervisors to be able to demonstrate excellence in both mentoring and monitoring for supervision to function effectively and be rooted in a relational ethic.

Hawkins and Shohet (2000) suggested that supervision holds the supervisee's helping relationship within a 'therapeutic triad' that enables them to continue to function effectively in a professional helping relationship. They considered that this necessitates an integration of the roles of educator, supporter and manager through a relationship-based approach. Stratton and

Hanks (2016, p. 7) proposed that 'all forms of training and personal professional development are fundamentally learning'. They considered that to facilitate this, supervision must necessarily be based in andragogy (theories of adult learning).

Cullen (2017) proposed that systemic supervision was based on four compass points: ethics, experience, literature and knowledge. She suggested that these concepts might form a sort of weathervane that is not static and enables a both/and position in the use of the four points of supervision.

Figure 14.1 shows a model of themes and commitments in a proposed systemic supervision approach that is adapted from Williams and Watson's (1988) feminist (power) analysis of family therapy; Carr's (2006) themes of family therapy; and Beinart's (2012) tasks of supervision.

Carr (2006) considers that the various schools of systemic approaches tend towards a therapeutic focus in their pursuit of one of three themes: problem-maintaining behaviour patterns; the family members' belief systems, scripts and narratives that support the maintenance of the behaviour; and the wider historical and social contexts that led to those belief systems and narratives. These themes are equally useful and applicable in a supervisory context. Additionally, they resonate with the focus that Dallos and Draper

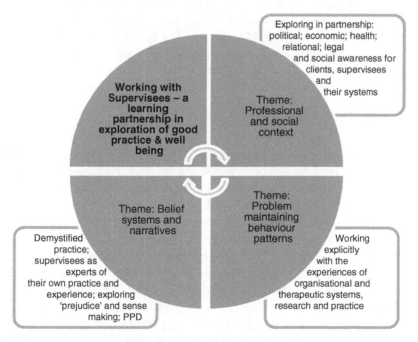

Figure 14.1   Proposed themes and commitments in a systemic supervision approach

Adapted from Carr (2006); Williams and Watson (1988); Beinart (2012)

(2005) accord to feminist systemic practitioners' attention to the individual, the relationship and the wider social context. They cite Williams and Watson (1988) who emphasise the importance of these foci through the use of three 'core commitments' in feminist practice: equality within therapy; bringing the social context into therapy; and power redistribution in society. These are arguably just as relevant to the nature of supervision: AFT (Association for Family Therapy and Systemic Practice in the United Kingdom, 2016) specify that supervision should be collaborative, which requires a mutual respect and recognition of second-order working; Burnham (e.g. 1993, 2005) highlights the need for supervision to be relationally reflexive; and critical awareness of the role of power in training and supervision was specifically highlighted by Flaskas (2014). This is represented in Figure 14.1.

The idea of supervisees as experts of their own practice draws parallels with the work of Paulo Freire, who said 'you never get there by starting from there, you get there by starting from some here ... the educator must not be ignorant of, underestimate, or reject any of the "knowledge of experience" with which educands come' (1994, p. 49).

Supervisors focusing on creating a learning process are therefore challenged to explore what their supervisees bring to supervision – this is a clear link with systemic ideas about considering one's own prejudices (Cecchin et al., 1994) and epistemologies (theories and ideas that inform your practice). Indeed, Vetere et al. (2016) suggest that it is this emphasis on 'pattern and process' and 'context and meaning' that 'defines' systemic practice and arguably, therefore, systemic supervision.

Methods of systemic supervision

This principally concerns the context in which supervision happens. This aspect of supervision is often where both the supervisor and the supervisee may have limited influence because it is likely to be guided by organisational norms and existing patterns of working. For example, it might include consideration of individual or group approaches; in-house or independent supervision; contracted and paid for by the supervisee or the employer; known or unknown supervisors; selected by the individual or appointed by a service manager. Flaskas (2014) acknowledged that 'different teaching and learning contexts allow and demand different conditions' and that this would apply equally to different professional and practice contexts.

Despite considerable multidisciplinary agreement about the importance of supervision to promote good practice (Senediak, 2013) there are often wildly varying professional requirements for continuing professional development and supervision. Thus in some fields supervision and dedicated time are highly valued, although it is unclear whether they are professionally required. For example, practitioner psychologists must understand the importance of participating in supervision as well as different ways of doing it but there is no specific requirement to attend supervision in order to stay registered with the Health and Care Professions Council (HCPC, 2015). In other professions, whilst a strong personal tutor/supervisory relationship is a tenet of training, there is no post-qualifying enforcement of probationary mentoring arrangements (e.g. nursing). When supervision is not required it can easily become diminished or undervalued, particularly as resources become squeezed.

A key consideration in the context of the supervision process is drawing up a contract or agreement that clearly delineates clinical responsibility and lines of accountability (AFT, 2016). This incorporates who is paying for the arrangements, issues of indemnity and liability, and recording and reporting arrangements. There are the same concerns in professional higher education for first-level qualifying courses, for example nursing, psychology and social work, which require considerable multi-agency negotiation and clear flow charts and communication regarding clinical, academic and personal development and support for students. There should also be specific arrangements for recording, reporting and raising concerns that come to light in a supervision context (AFT, 2016).

Methods for monitoring the outcomes of supervision are also an important consideration. There are increasingly a wide range of tools and theories that can be used and adapted to create frameworks for this purpose. However, it is important to note that each tool will reflect different approaches and methods of supervision and have more or less relevance in a given context. For example, the Supervisory Working Alliance Inventory (Efstation et al., 1990) highlights that it is founded in an approach that prioritises the relational aspects of supervisory relationships and the common factors of therapeutic relationships. This was also the focus in Wainwright's (2010) Leeds Alliance in Supervision Scale.

Box 14.1 Reflective questions on supervision

- What sort of supervision methods have you been offered?

- Who was the best supervisor you ever had? What was it about them and how they supervised you that makes them stick out in your memory? What approach, method and techniques did they use?

- If you were to write a person specification for a new supervisor, what skills, knowledge and attributes would you be looking for?

Techniques of systemic supervision and reflection

Arguably, it is the activity of relational reflection and reflexivity (e.g. Burnham, 1993, 2005) that distinguishes systemic reflection and supervision from the generally self-oriented reflective models adopted by many professions. For example Gibbs' (1988) reflective cycle considers the description, feelings, evaluation, analysis and conclusion of an event, but only through the eyes of the person reflecting. Similarly, Johns' evolving model of reflection (2017) guides us to consider aesthetics, personal, ethics, and empirics, but what of the inter- and intra-personal issues that are fundamental to any moment between two human beings? Interestingly, Johns' most recent 17th edition of his model guides reflectors to consider the factors that influenced the way that they responded. Included here are the expectations of others and self 'about how I should act' and also about how others were feeling (2017, p. 38). Yet even these considerations are in relation to the actions of the reflector rather than what it is that they and the other person are making together and in what way the actions of the reflector may have influenced the other person(s). Burnham (1993) considered self-reflexivity as a process of reflecting on action in order to 'recalibrate' how we act in relation to others, whilst relational reflexivity entails 'talking about talking': it is a willingness to engage collaboratively with a person in order to 'consider, explore, experiment with and elaborate with ways in which they relate' (Burnham, 2005, p. 4). These are key considerations in both supervision and practice; I would argue especially so when with people whose voice, position and power have been as systematically challenged as they have been for men and women labelled with learning disabilities. See the section on relational reflexivity in Chapter 28 for more on its practical application.

The similarities between therapy and supervision generate considerable discussion (McCarthy, 2010); however, it is generally recognised that they offer very distinct relationships due to having different boundaries, goals and functions (AFT, 2016). There is, however, there is sufficient similarity in the two activities that techniques used in a therapeutic context can be usefully modelled and utilised in the context of a supervisory relationship – thus any paper that explores a specific technique, and indeed method or approach, in systemic therapy can become a useful and creative resource in the context of supervision. The key consideration is to ensure that the supervisor and supervisee are both aware of the intentionality of the activity and have considered the likely effect on the individual or group. A challenge in any form of training or supervision context is to ensure that the learning opportunities (techniques) offered are likely to facilitate learning that will have the best impact on the supervisees' competence and confidence. The choice of activity should take into account the supervisee's stage of training, professional practice and previous experience. It is also important to factor in ongoing feedback about what is working well and what is not working to avoid the supervisory relationship becoming ineffective or possibly even unsafe. Thus it is through an alchemy of group and individual learning theories (e.g. Vygotsky, 1978; Schön, 1983; Lave & Wenger, 1991; hooks, 1994) and systemic therapeutic techniques that supervisors and supervisees can come together to create and experiment with a varied range of systemic supervisory techniques.

There is an extremely wide and ever-increasing range of edited texts (e.g. Holloway, 1995; Campbell & Mason, 2002; Moon, 2004; Stirk & Sanderson, 2012; Bownas & Fredman, 2016; Vetere & Stratton, 2016) that offer a multitude of systemically oriented techniques that can promote Flaskas' three Rs and systemic thinking. For example, Senediak (2013) highlights a range of strategies that can be utilised to support supervisees in a training context to learn and practise the reflective skill of considering the thinking and theories behind their actions and communication in an interaction with a client. This supervision can be live (being supervised in the moment) or retrospective (looking back on it afterwards) and might incorporate inviting them to collaborate on family-of-origin work or explore a critical incident in their practice experience. These techniques have the potential to enhance our capacity to identify our own experiences and needs and also prepare us to respond more effectively to people, families or colleagues in similar situations in the future.

Faris (2002) recounted the approach used in my own qualifying training programme, to teach a group meta-communication through an experiential personal and professional development group. At the time I found the process excruciatingly painful and frustrating, and yet looking back I can see that many of the learning goals intended were indeed achieved in terms of increasing my skills in analysing and reflecting on group process, as well as enhancing my understanding of changing definitions of relationship.

However, for the remainder of this brief chapter I am going to focus on two techniques that I believe are specifically relevant to supervision in the context of working with systems that include people with learning disabilities whose voices are frequently diminished by the systems around them.

Haydon-Laurelut et al. (2012) outline an 'AS IF' technique that is useful in supervision with teams of more than three. It is designed to create a new opportunity for conversation in complex systems. 'AS IF' invites practitioners consulting on a complicated issue to become listeners to a conversation between an interviewer and an interviewee. One, or more if it is a big group, listener is allocated a specific person who is significant in the system. This could be the person labelled with learning disability, their

mother, father, nan, social worker, service manager, nurse or even a neighbour if they are a key part of the system and the practitioner's dilemma.
The 'AS IF' listeners then actively listen to the interviewer and interviewee
as they discuss the case and specific dilemma 'AS IF' they are listening as
the person they have been allocated. Particular attention in this 'listened to'
interview is given to the relational connections between the people in the
system. Haydon-Laurelut et al. (2012) suggested the following questions for
the interview:

What do we need to know in order to be useful in this conversation?

Who is in conversation in this issue?

Who is most concerned about this issue?

Who sees this differently?

How have you responded so far, who do you talk to, what do you do and say?

What would you be most interested to hear from the listeners?

The listeners are then invited to feed back to each other their experience of
listening 'AS IF' they are the person they were allocated. They are asked to
use 'I' statements when they speak. In this way an 'AS IF' listener being the
person with a learning disability might comment: *'I don't understand what you
are all on about. Nobody is listening to me. Nobody is asking what I want!'*

Haydon-Laurelut et al. (2012) found that having followed this format for a
peer supervision, group participants subsequently reflected they had experienced their 'inner conversations' as 'outer conversations' which enabled them
to:

➢ feel less stuck,

➢ create new ideas about possible next steps,

➢ hear the voice of the person with learning disabilities,

➢ identify emotions in the system so that they could acknowledge and
respond to them more effectively,

➢ have a new and more empathic understanding of the individuals in the
system,

➢ listen to the views of others in a non-defensive way.

This process of bringing internal conversations, the thoughts and dialogue
that we have with ourselves in our head, into spoken dialogue with others

can also be achieved using a process called 'internalised other interviewing' that Parè (2001) suggests was developed by a number of practitioners. One person is interviewed, again with a focus on relational questions (how do you get on and make sense of each other), and they are asked to answer in the first person using their own ideas about how a named other person might respond. The interviewer will use the name of the person they are considering as if it were that person sitting in front of them. Tomm (1999) suggested that in order to do this they rely on their own 'inner experience' of the other person's 'inner experience' and speaking this aloud can be enough to create the potential for change in their relationship. The interview can be done with just one person or it can include the internalised other person actually in the room as a listener. If the latter is the case, it is important to ask the other person if there were answers that had been a good fit for them and if there were responses they felt reflected misunderstandings. This technique can offer a powerful opportunity to attend to the voices of people with learning disabilities who might otherwise not be included (Haydon-Laurelut & Wilson (2011) explain the technique in more detail). It is not an alternative to trying to establish a person's views directly but it can aid this process when people have been thoughtfully prepared. This includes considering the support that interviewees may require if they truly succeed in gaining new insight into the inner experiences of a person whose voice, for whatever reason, has been diminished, as this has the potential to be a difficult experience. This process of 'interviewing an internalised other' has the potential to make changes in a relationship by helping us to focus on how we understand and make sense of it.

If we return, then, to the original question regarding what it is that makes supervision systemic we can conclude that it is a joint endeavour in the pursuit of reflection, recursivity and both self and relational reflexivity in order to achieve better practice in human services. Each supervisory relationship and encounter is necessarily embedded in a combination of approach, method and technique. When a supervisory conversation promotes learning and better practice in an ethical, relational, reflexive and recursive frame it becomes systemic supervision, regardless of the context or profession of the supervisees.

References

Association for Family Therapy and Systemic Practice in the United Kingdom (AFT) (2009). *The Red Book*. www.aft.org.uk/SpringboardWebApp/userfiles/aft/file/Training/RED%20BOOK%20April%202009%20final.pdf (accessed 20 September 2017).

Association for Family Therapy and Systemic Practice in the United Kingdom (AFT) (2011). *Code of Ethics and Practice for Supervisors*. www.aft.org.uk/SpringboardWebApp/userfiles/aft/file/Members/Supervision/Code%20of%20Ethics%20and%20Practice%20for%20Supervisors%202012.pdf (accessed 20 September 2017), published by AFT, London.

Association for Family Therapy and Systemic Practice in the United Kingdom (AFT) (2016). *Supervision information sheet*. www.aft.org.uk/SpringboardWebApp/userfiles/aft/file/Information%20Sheets/Supervision%20Information%20Sheet%20Dec%202016.pdf (accessed 20 September 2017).

Beinart, H. (2012). Clinical supervision and wellbeing. DCP annual conference 2012. Oxford Institute of Clinical Psychology Training.

Bownas, J. & Fredman, G. (eds) (2016). *Working with Embodiment in Supervision*. London: Routledge.

Burnham, J. (1993). Systemic supervision: The evolution of reflexivity in the context of the supervisory relationship. *Human Systems*, 4, 349–381.

Burnham, J. (2005). Relational reflexivity: A tool for socially constructing therapeutic relationships. In C. Flaskas, B. Mason & A. Perlesz, (eds) *The Space Between* (pp. 1–18). London: Karnac Books.

Burns, R. (1786). To a Louse, *Poems, Chiefly in the Scottish Dialect*. Printed by John Wilson. www.bl.uk/learning/timeline/item126722.html (accessed 25 February 2018).

Campbell, D. & Mason, B. (eds) (2002). *Perspectives on Supervision*. London: Karnac.

Carr, A. (2006). *Family Therapy Concepts, Process and Practice*. 2nd edition. Chichester: Wiley and Sons.

Cecchin, G., Lane, G. & Ray, W.A. (1994). *The Cybernetics of Prejudices in the Practice of Psychotherapy*. London: Karnac.

Cullen, N. (2017). Signposts and weathercocks: Travels with ethics in supervision practice in Hull. *Context*, 152, 4–7.

Dallos, R. & Draper, R. (2005). *An Introduction to Family Therapy*. 3rd edition. Maidenhead: McGraw Hill.

Dallos, R. & Stedmon, J. (2009). Flying over the swampy lowlands: Reflective and reflexive Practice. In R. Dallos & J. Stedmon (eds), *Reflective Practice in Psychotherapy and Counselling* (pp. 1–22). Milton Keynes: Open University Press.

Efstation, J., Kardash, C.A., Patton, M. (1990). Measuring the Working Alliance in Counselor Supervision. *Journal of Counseling Psychology*, 37(3), 322–329

Faris, J. (2002). Some reflections on process, relationship, and personal development in supervision. In D. Campbell & B. Mason (eds), *Perspectives on Supervision* (pp. 91–112). London: Karnac.

Flaskas, C. (2014). Teaching and learning theory for family therapy practice: On the art and craft of balancing. *Australian and New Zealand Journal of Family Therapy*, 34, 283–293.

Freire, P. (1994). *Pedagogy of Hope*. London: Bloomsbury Revelations.

Gibbs, G. (1988). *Learning by Doing: A Guide to Teaching and Learning Methods.* Oxford: Oxford Further Education Unit.

Hawkins, P. & Shohet, R. (2000). *Supervision in the Helping Professions an Individual, Group and Organizational Approach.* 2nd edition. Milton Keynes: Open University Press.

Haydon-Laurelut, M., Millett, E., Bissmire, D., Doswell, S. & Heneage, C. (2012). It helps to untangle really complicated situations: 'AS IF' supervision for working with complexity. *Clinical Psychology & People with Learning Disabilities Special Edition: Systemic Approaches,* 10(2), 26–32.

Haydon-Laurelut, M. & Wilson, C. (2011). Interviewing the internalized other. *Journal of Systemic Therapies,* 30(1), 24–37.

Health and Care Professions Council (HCPC). (2015). *Standards of Proficiency Practitioner Psychologists.* London: HCPC.

Holloway, E. (1995). *Clinical Supervision a Systems Approach.* London: Sage.

hooks, b. (1994). *Teaching to Transgress.* London: Routledge.

Johns, C. (2017). *Becoming a Reflective Practitioner.* 5th edition. Chichester: John Wiley and Sons Ltd.

Lave, J. & Wenger, E. (1991). *Situated Learning Legitimate Peripheral Participation.* Cambridgeshire: Cambridge University Press.

McCarthy, I. (2010). Fifth Province Diamonds: Contrasts in coordinated play. http://imeldamccarthy.webmate.me/Publications_and_Downloads_files/Fifth%20 Province%20Diamonds%20for%20Supervision.pdf (accessed 25 February 2019).

Moon, J. (2004). *A Handbook of Reflective and Experiential Learning; Theory and Practice.* London: Routledge Falmer.

Paré, D.A. (2001). Crossing the Divide: The Therapeutic use of internalized other interviewing. *Journal of Activities in Psychotherapy Practice,* 1(4), 21–28.

Schön, D. (1983). *The Reflective Practitioner: How Professionals Think in Action.* London: Temple Smith.

Senediak, C. (2013). Integrating reflective practice in family therapy supervision. *Australian and New Zealand Journal of Family Therapy,* 34(4), 338–351.

Shaw, E. (2013). Mentoring or monitoring: Formulating a balance in systemic supervision. *Australian and New Zealand Journal of Family Therapy,* 34(4), 296–310.

Somerville, D. & Keeling, J. (2004). A practical approach to promote reflective practice within nursing. *Nursing Times,* 100(12), 42–45.

Stirk, S. & Sanderson, H. (2012). *Creating Person-Centred Organisations; Strategies and Tools for Managing Change in Health, Social Care and the Voluntary Sector.* London: Jessica Kingsley Publishers.

Stratton, P. & Hanks, H. (2016). PPD as processes of learning that enable the practitioner to create a self that is equipped for higher levels of professional mastery. In A. Vetere & P. Stratton (eds), *Interacting Selves* (pp. 7–32). London: Routledge.

Tate, S. & Sills, M. (2004). *The Development of Critical Reflection in the Health Professions.* London: Higher Education Academy.

Tomm, K. (1999). Co-Constructing Responsibility. In S. McNamee & K.J. Gergen (eds), *Relational Responsibility* (pp.129–37). London: Sage Publications Ltd.

Vetere, A., Stratton, P., Hanks, H., Jensen, P., Protopsalti-Polychroni, K. & Sheehan, J. (2016). Chapter one prologue and introduction to the systemic approach to personal and professional development. In A. Vetere & P. Stratton (eds), *Interacting Selves*, (pp. 1–6). London: Routledge

Vetere, A. & Stratton, P.E. (2016). *Interacting Selves*. London: Routledge.

Vygotsky, L.S. (1978). *Mind in Society: The Development of Higher Psychological Processes*. Cambridge, MA: Harvard University Press.

Wainwright, N. (2010). *The Development of the Leeds Alliance in Supervision Scale*. Unpublished D.Clin.Psych. thesis, University of Leeds.

Williams, J.A. & Watson, G. (1988) Sexual inequality, family life and family therapy. In E. Street & W. Dryden (eds) (1988). *Family therapy in Britain*. Psychotherapy in Britain series. Milton Keynes: Open University Press.

15

Evidence-Based Practice and Practice-Based Evidence

Victoria Jones and Mark Haydon-Laurelut

Accessible summary

- Knowing what works well can help us to make good decisions. This can be called *evidence-based practice*.

- Finding out about things is called research. Research can be about what works well for lots of people or about what people think about something.

- To help people with learning disabilities to make good decisions there does not need to be special research that is just for them. Their bodies, feelings and experiences are human just like everyone else.

- Staff whose job is to help people to have a good life need to be able to understand research studies and to know whether a study is useful or not.

- Trying things out over time and finding out what works well for each person is also really important. This can be called *practice-based evidence.*

- Practice-based evidence can be especially important for people who do not have speech – the wisdom of experts by experience needs to be recorded and used.

- Even when there is research that says something is brilliant and the best thing to do, we need to remember that it may not be right for everyone. This is how we make sure that our practice is person-centred.

Health and social care professionals in the twenty-first century are generally encouraged to operate from a scientific, knowledge-based perspective and use evidence-based practice (EBP). Sackett et al. (1996) identified 'three pillars' of EBP: the best research evidence, clinical expertise and patient values/

preferences in the pursuit of a good decision. One of the challenges of this approach to identifying the best way forward for someone, or good professional decision making, is the assumption that what needs to be known is all in the control of the expert professional. In Western professional culture we tend to prioritise science over preferences, and thus the contribution of the individual themselves becomes at risk of being viewed merely as a fussy annoyance.

Trevithick (2008) distinguished between three different ways we can know about something: theoretically, factually (including research) and practically/personally. However, a crucial difference between her approach to EBP and that of Sackett et al. (1996) is that she specifically includes and recognises the knowledge of service users and carers as key contributions to what is known alongside that of any professionals in the system. Indeed, if we are to work collaboratively and co-productively then it is necessary, when exploring a decision or dilemma, to draw from the existing concepts, ideas and resources in the entire system and ensure that the techne (skills and artistry), episteme (scientific and theoretical knowledge) and nous (intuitive intelligence) of every part of the system are recognised, utilised and celebrated. It is particularly important when we are supporting people who may not use language and may have multiple impairments to ensure that the practical wisdom (phronesis) of the people who know them well is included in the information that we collect and rely on to promote their wellbeing.

Additionally, Messmer and Hitzler (2008) suggest that we need to consider the process of how we act as well as what it is we intend to do as part of EBP. They propose that this requires that we are not limited to only considering a 'top-down view' but that we also include a 'bottom-up framework'. This approach connects with exploring the relational reflexivity (Burnham, 1993) of our interactions and processes. These factors can be a useful focus of research.

To be able to advocate for the best outcomes for the people we serve, professionals need to be able to find out and understand what is considered to be the gold standard in their area of practice. Arguably, then, we all have a duty to acquire the skills and confidence necessary to access and make use of research. A vital part of professional expertise is the ability to supply information and perform our role in ways that are considered to be optimally effective. However, professionals also need to be able to synthesise all the different ways of knowing a person, their system and context in order to ensure that people with learning disabilities have access to truly collaborative and person-centred opportunities to make the best decisions.

A systemic approach recognises this best-outcomes approach to EBP through its focus on mobilising the existing resources in a system to make change possible. Rather than focusing on what caused a situation there is more of an emphasis on what might be making it hard to resolve and how everyone in a family, staff team or human system might benefit both now and in the future from a different way of making sense of it all.

Stratton (2016) undertook a review of the evidence base of family therapy and systemic practice. He concluded that there is a significant amount of evidence to support the efficacy of systemic therapy as an approach. He cites the work of Retzlaff et al. (2013), Sydow et al. (2010) and Guo & Slesnick (2013) as evidence of the benefits of systemic therapy for children, families and adults with a wide range of referred needs.

Indeed, Stratton was able to distinguish 72 'conditions' (40 in children and 32 in adults) that have positive evidence for the efficacy of a systemic approach. Whilst it is notable, and perhaps quite proper, that 'learning disability' itself does not appear on this list, many of the concerns of individuals, their families and systems that do appear might be familiar to professionals working in the field. For example: ADHD; anxiety; Asperger's; attachment; behavioural difficulties; child abuse and neglect; couple discord; depression; encopresis; enuresis; feeding difficulties; personal social systems; poor emotional regulation; relational autonomy; relationship distress; self-esteem and self-acceptance; self-harm; sleep difficulties; and substance misuse (Stratton, 2016).

Stratton reminds us that available evidence is often merely a reflection of social concerns and research funding priorities and suggests that it is important to remember that a '[l]ack of evidence of effectiveness is not evidence of ineffectiveness' (2016, p. 11).

Research is an area where human service professionals need to advocate for change, for example through seeking funds for good quality studies that explore the specific needs of people with learning disabilities; recognising that people labelled with a learning disability are a heterogeneous group who have as much in common with the rest of the population as each other; or supporting opportunities for people with learning disabilities to be participants in a wide range of generic research studies. It is also vital to ensure that future research projects recognise that people with learning disabilities have ideas for research and should be involved at every stage of a research project if we are to ensure that our evidence base is holistic and effectively draws from what is known in *all* the ways that we can know something.

Miss Lynne Evans summed this up in the speech she gave when she became an Honorary Fellow of the University of South Wales for her leadership and contribution to participatory research, self-advocacy and the rights of people with learning disabilities in Wales:

> Like the Welsh football team I believe that together we are stronger.

> It is important that we all work together as a team and know that everyone has something valuable to give.

When we all work together we can make stronger communities and better patient care.

I am very proud to be part of a University where this is really happening.

(Graduation Ceremony, July 2016)

Systemic approaches attend to issues of power. This is particularly relevant in research where knowledge can be considered a form of power and the ability to define the question, that is to decide what is researched, how and by whom, could be considered an ultimate form of power (Lukes, 2005).

Lannamann invites us to notice the things that limit our choices and actions, recognise our discomfort, question what might be considered 'taken for granted' knowledge or expertise, and celebrate our curiosity in the pursuit of new knowledge that can be useful and effective for individuals. This creates potential for a shift in power relations.

> When we see the constraints that limit our choices we are aware of power relations; When we see only choices we live in and reproduce power ... The potential of ideo-logical analysis is that it decenters the powerful assumptions that determine our questions.

> Lannamann (1991, p. 198)

Box 15.1 Reflective questions on knowledge and power

- Have you ever heard a phrase like 'This would be a great/easy job if it wasn't for the clients'? What might this sort of statement suggest about the way that clients, collaboration and power are perceived in this service?

- What criteria do you employ to understand the success of a piece of work? Whose voices are centred and whose are marginalised by these criteria?

- With whom are the outcomes (and processes) of your work shared? With whom might it be important to share this knowledge?

Warm data

Data can be 'big', but did you know it can also be 'warm' (or cold)? With the concept of warm data we may remind ourselves of the interrelationality and multiple contextuality of life. There are many ways to experience, make sense of and describe the world. Data, evidence and knowledge more generally can be experienced, gathered and represented in multiple ways. Bateson (2016), who began using this term, notes, for example:

> At a recent session on Big Data I got a super-sized tummy ache. It appears to be the beanstalk sprouted from quantitative magic beans and binary rain. Huge scoops of numbers get formed into patterns, and then, good heavens, and then we call it information ... The thing about numbers is that they pretend to be 'objective,' they carry a tone of 'facts and figures' when in fact they are objectifying and much more slippery in the stories they carry than poetry.

(Bateson, 2016, p. 105)

Warm data does not replace detailed understanding of specific aspects of practice, of a referral difficulty, health condition and so on; however, it directs us to consider the multiple contexts, multiple voices, and the systemic interdependence of persons and ideas-in-context.

In order to create warmth in our data it is not enough to capture multiple perspectives:

> Warm Data is about the transcontextual 'relational' information. Many people try to use systems thinking by streaming in different kinds of data ... from multiple perspectives. And, sadly they think this will give them systemic information. But it doesn't. Why? Because what gives the system its vitality (no matter what we think of it) is the relationship between the perspectives. No amount of multiplicity will actually give you that. So the warmth is warm precisely because it addresses the relational realms that give a complex system its integrity.

(Bateson, 2018)

Perspectives rub up against, influence, constrain and create contexts for each other. Mutual learning and interdependence are involved.

Box 15.2 A reflective question about warm data

Consider a piece of work you have been involved in and ask yourself: how is the relationship between different sources, or perspectives, of information and data about a person, or a piece of research, explored and recorded?

Rather than a static drawing together of perspectives, we are encouraged to consider the living ecology of beliefs, language, and other practices in which our lives take place.

One important aspect of the 'warmth' of data is the manner in which it represents a life, as Bateson (2016, p. 162) notes: 'It is not difficult to see that delivery of data in graphs depicting statistical breakdown of the gathered information implies a methodology. What is not so obvious is the meta-message that life is clear and definable.' Is this how you experience life? This has myriad consequences. One may be that when we are working with complexity – with people and their lives and the difficulties they face – the delivery and beliefs and ideas about data may present a powerful meta-message about these people's lives and our work with them. It may describe who can be a knower (the person with a learning disability or the professional that collected data and produced a graph?) and what kind of knowing should be possible (we should be clear about what is going on and be able to define it). The power of some kinds of data and its delivery (e.g. the use of statistics, PowerPoint presentations, graphs and so on) is not only in what it tells us but how it tells us and how it builds its credibility by, for example, its drawing on the modes of representation of science. We might hear that the stories of those we support, their families and networks and our own experiences are 'just' anecdotal, that we need some 'hard' or even perhaps some 'big(ger)' data. Phenomenological knowledge (the knowledge from experience) and relational knowledge (the understandings that we develop between ourselves and others in a community) may be seen as invalid if this kind of data becomes too dominant in a context. Person-centred practices and practice-based evidence can be powerful responses to this.

Box 15.3 Reflective questions on evidence, knowledge and power

Consider the following questions for a piece of work you have been involved in – you might consider sharing them with others involved, too:

Whose ideas are most powerful in this situation?

What kinds of data – stories, experiences, numbers, graphs – are privileged?

How is data being delivered? In a presentation by a professional? As the process of a discussion between the person and those in their network? In the sharing of a story the person with learning disability wishes to tell?

What meta-message is sent in the way in which data is presented?

To restate the question above: *How is the relationship between different sources, or perspectives, of information and data about a person, or a piece of research, explored and recorded?*

What other ways of co-creating knowledge together can be created here? How might we together come to know differently?

References

Bateson, N. (2016). *Small Arcs of Larger Circles, Framing through Other Patterns.* England: Triarchy Press.

Bateson, N. (2018). Personal communication with Haydon-Laurelut, M.

Burnham, J. (1993). Systemic supervision: the evolution of reflexivity in the context of the supervisory relationship. *Human Systems*, 4(19), 349–381.

Guo, X. & Slesnick, N. (2013). Family versus individual therapy: Impact on discrepancies between parents' and adolescents' perceptions over time. *Journal of Marital and Family Therapy*, 39, 182–194.

Lannamann, J.W. (1991). Interpersonal communication research as ideological practice. *Communication Theory*, 1(3), 179–203.

Lukes, S. (2005). *Power A Radical View*, 2nd edition. Basingstoke: Palgrave Macmillan.

Messmer, H. & Hitzler, S. (2008). Practice-based evidence – Social work practice viewed from an interaction perspective. In I. Bryderup (ed.), *Evidence Based and Knowledge Based Social Work* (pp. 33–52). Denmark: Aarhus University Press.

Retzlaff, R., Sydow, K., Beher, S., Haun, M. & Schweitzer, J. (2013). The efficacy of systemic therapy for internalizing and other disorders of childhood and adolescence: A systematic review of 38 randomized trials. *Family Process*, 52(4), 619–652.

Sackett D, Rosenberg W, Gray J, Haynes R, Richardson W. Evidence based medicine: what it is and what it isn't. *BMJ* 1996; 312: 71

Stratton, P. (2016). *The Evidence Base of Family Therapy and Systemic Practice.* United Kingdom: The Association for Family Therapy and Systemic Practice.

Sydow, K., Beher, S., Schweitzer, J. & Retzlaff, R. (2010). The efficacy of systemic therapy with adult patients: A meta-content analysis of 38 randomized controlled trials. *Family Process*, 49(4), 653–672.

Trevithick, P. (2008). Revisiting the knowledge base of social work: A framework for practice. *British Journal of Social Work*, 38, 1212–1237.

Note

1   See also this short clip of Nora Bateson discussing Warm Data: www.youtube.com/watch?v=cRjv4wzuBWQ.

Section III

Introduction: Working Systemically When You are Not a Qualified Family Therapist

Victoria Jones and Mark Haydon-Laurelut

As we have seen, systemic thinking and practice extends far beyond the therapy room. A systemic approach foregrounds the relational aspects of our worlds. We can all think about context, story, pattern, and be curious and have a commitment to work collaboratively. Using tools that have the potential to improve human interaction and enhance communication with people with learning disabilities is something that we should all strive for. This third section of the book is a reference toolkit containing a range of systemic techniques and practices with a brief exploration of their specific relevance and application in systems that include people with learning disabilities. Each mini-chapter briefly highlights a specific tool, exercise, activity or technique that has its roots in systemic approaches with examples of ways in which it can be used collaboratively to create change. It is important to highlight that this is not a guide on how to do family and systemic therapy with people with learning disabilities, or anyone else. However, these are tools that you might come across if you ever do attend for a family therapy session or systemic consultation.

In exploring what it is that makes a conversation therapeutic rather than 'merely' a communication, Anderson and Goolishian (1988) suggest that a therapeutic system is one where the communication has a relevance specific to itself. Bertrando (2007) reflects this view in the suggestion that it is the therapeutic frame that makes a conversation therapeutic. However, Tomm observes that every question we ever ask of clients or colleagues is effectively an intervention, as they will respond to the query and it will impact upon the way we 'do' being in relationship and communication together (Tomm, 1987). So whilst we are, in Tomm's sense, intervening at the point at which we ask a question, we are not necessarily doing this in the context of a therapeutic relationship.

Considerations for engaging with Section 3 of this book

➢ Systemic techniques are not practices that we do to people; they are rather conversations or activities that we invite people to participate in. Consent is crucial. Contemporary systemic practice eschews practising in secret. We aim for transparency in our practices. We talk with those who consult us about what we might do together. When engaging in this section of the book, make sure that you are acting *with* people, not *for* them or *to* them.

➢ Ensure that you have team support or it is possible that you are setting yourself up to fail.

➢ Make good use of supervision. This can be managerial, clinical, mentoring or peer support, but having a focused window to debrief and think aloud about the process and outcomes of your systemic practice is critical.

➢ Warm the context. It is usually best not to leap straight into an activity but take time to make sure everyone knows why they are here, what the goals are, and that they are prepared for what is coming next.

➢ Self-reflexivity. It is important that we pay attention to how it is we are using any form of practice, how we feel, what our intention is and what effect our actions may be having on others. Are we especially attached to a particular idea, outcome, or system member's viewpoint? Are we able to maintain our curiosity? When are we less able to do this and how might this influence the client?

➢ Domains of production. The domains (Lang et al., 1990) help us to be clear about when we are exploring meanings and narrative with our clients (the domain of explanation); when we have external, perhaps legal or professional duties that we must speak to, such as safeguarding (the domain of production); and how we move between these contexts in a manner that enables useful work to continue (the domain of aesthetics).

➢ Recording. As with all of our work we need to make sure that we have a secure and confidential space to store any items that are co-produced as part of an activity. Be clear about who owns them.

If you are interested in using these techniques as a systemic and family therapist please refer to the end of the book where there is a section which signposts how to find out about training to become a systemic and family therapist.

References

Anderson, H. & Goolishian, H. (1988). Human systems as linguistic systems: Evolving ideas for the implications in theory and practice. *Family Process, 27,* 371–393.

Bertrando, P. (2007). *The Dialogical Therapist.* London: Karnac Books.

Lang, P., Little, M. & Cronen, V. (1990). The systemic professional: Domains of action and the question of neutrality. *Human Systems, 1,* 39–55.

Tomm, K. (1987). Interventive interviewing: Part 1. Strategizing as a fourth guideline for the therapist. *Family Process, 26(1),* Mar, 3–13.

16

Ascribed Roles

Victoria Jones

Accessible summary

- Through history, groups of people who are not valued by society have been given parts to play in their community.

- These parts are called *roles*.

- Roles are still important today.

- Being given a role can often have a bad effect on people, what they can do and the kinds of services that they have.

- Roles affect the way that we think we can work with and for people.

It is nearly 50 years since Wolfensberger (1972) proposed that society ascribes (or allocates) roles to those it considers deviant. He suggested that we do this largely to be able to manage groups of people who are considered to be different in a way that is negatively valued. Ideas about what constitutes deviance are socially constructed and vary across cultures, communities and time. A good example of this can be seen in attitudes to sexuality and sexual orientation over the last 60 years. Groups of people who might be considered to be 'deviant' or devalued by society today might include (but are not limited to) the homeless; refugees; travellers; asylum seekers; the unemployed; and disabled people, particularly those with learning disability. Wolfensberger proposed that throughout history all people who have been considered deviant in some way have been managed by dominant groups through being ascribed specific social roles; namely, the 'deviant' individual is perceived as:

➤ A subhuman organism

➤ A menace

➤ An unspeakable object of dread

➤ An object of pity

➤ A holy innocent

➤ A diseased organism

➤ An object of ridicule

➤ An eternal child

At first glance it could be very easy to look at this list and consider that it may have historical significance, but does not really have much to add to our practice in the twenty-first century.

Table 16.1 identifies examples of the impact upon people with learning disabilities of being ascribed these social roles across history and, crucially, how they often remain part of our thinking and actions today. Table 16.1 also demonstrates how ascribed roles impact upon language and service models. For example, if we think that someone is less than human it becomes possible to end their life without being a murderer (eugenics). If someone is an object of ridicule it is possible to make a programme about their struggle to find a life partner and call it factual entertainment which makes you laugh (*The Undateables*, Betty Production Co., 2012– present). It is possible to see the interplay between these ascribed roles and different types of service, language and conversations and how they contribute to the experiences of living with a learning disability today. Wolfensberger's ascribed roles show both historical impact and current potential to affect lives and outcomes for women, men and children with learning disability. Consequently, it is vital that people working in services take time to consider the roles that we ourselves ascribe to the people that we support, as well as the more valued roles that we support them to aspire to and achieve.

Table 16.1 The impact of ascribed roles across time and contexts: services and approaches to people with learning disability

Ascribed Role	Terminology and language	Service agency	Model of provision	Example	Modern legacy
Eternal child	'He'll never grow up' 'She thinks like a child'	The State Education	Protection and paternalism	Low expectations that people will gain employment or start a family	Legislation re. sexuality Day services that look like schools
Menace	Feeble-minded Moral imbecile Idiots Perverts	The State Penal/forensic	Segregation from society Institutional care	Enforced sterilisation Nazi extermination	'Not in my back yard' (NIMBY)
Object of dread	Lunatics Insane Danger to society 'Possessed by the devil'	Insane Should be 'kept in a locked room and have a keeper whom he fears' (Borde, 1542, cited by Tuke, 1882)	Incarceration and punishment	Chaining and whipping Demons cast out of 'possessed'	Ongoing fear and confusion regarding learning disability and mental health
Object of ridicule	Village idiot	Small rural Communities Entertainment industry	Theatre Travelling circus 'Freak show'	Court jester Quasimodo People with Down's Syndrome seen as happy	Playground use of: 'wally'; 'moron'; 'mong'; 'retard' Films like *The Waterboy* (Coraci, 1998); *The Ringer* (Blaustein, 2005)
Sick	Mentally ill Mentally handicapped Patients	The State Hospitals and asylums	Medical goal to 'make better'	Treatment e.g. electric shocks; blood letting Decisions based solely on medical risks	Learning disability nurses are the only professional group specifically trained to work with a group of people who are not unwell

Subhuman	'Cabbage' 'Changeling'	Unqualified, untrained and devalued staff	'Death making' and 'leaving to nature' 'All creatures great and small' at funerals of people with learning disability	Babies thought to be replaced by demons to punish parents	Late abortion if foetus is 'abnormal' Routine antenatal testing for Trisomy 21 (Down's Syndrome), high % of terminations when identified
Holy innocent	'Gift from God'	Charities and holy orders	Benevolence and paternalism 'Suffer little children'	Cretins in Switzerland seen as close to God Enable others to achieve virtue	'Doesn't know any better' and 'can do no wrong' attitudes
Object of pity and burden of charity	Burden 'Unfortunates' 'Handicap' (literally from 'cap in hand')	Charities and holy orders	Education and paternalism creating dependence	People seen as a drain on society and lucky recipients of care Enable others to achieve virtue	Children in Need/Comic Relief using images to raise funds Comments like 'You're so patient to work with those people. I don't know how you do it.'
New role: vulnerable person	Victim At risk Incompetent Lacks capacity Dependent and in need	Social services Police Service providers Parents and carers	Protectio Assessment of risk Investigation	People not supported to take risks Vulnerability is seen as in the person not their situation	
New role: citizen	Colleague Fellow peer	Legislature Service providers Communities Everyone	Promote rights, relationships and individuality	People recognised for their unique contribution to society Adequate support for a good life – financial, emotional and legal. Personalisation & co-production	

Incorporating: Wolfensberger, 1972; Stainton, 2008; Duffy & Perez, 2014.

It is also important to consider roles that have been added more recently and how they affect the way that we work with and for people today. For example, a key ascribed role for people with learning disabilities currently is that of *vulnerable person*. Services often tend to ascribe risk to the person 'because of' their learning disability rather than recognising that it is an environment, people and appropriate support that impact upon whether an individual is at risk in a *given context*. Thus we use language that focuses on risk and perceives people as weak and defenceless, requiring a multi-agency response that contains and mitigates those risks. This suggests that our professional role is to protect, take control and reduce risk. It makes possible paternalistic decisions that are not always entirely balanced, for example not dyeing a young man's greying hair just in case he has an anaphylactic reaction to the hair dye, or not supporting a person to go to a nightclub in case they meet someone who propositions them (for sex, drugs or something equally potentially 'risky').

Another social role more recently ascribed to people with learning disabilities is that of *citizen*. However, this role allocation is designed to claim equality rather than to mark people out as deviant. Indeed, Duffy and Perez (2014) consider that status as a citizen entails three things: equality; community; and recognition of difference. When we ascribe the role of citizen to those we support it would then follow that our role becomes to support individuals to defend their rights, have great relationships and celebrate all aspects of their uniqueness. Ascribed roles matter because they influence the way services are designed, the language we use, what is expected and what is possible.

An alternative to the idea of ascribed roles is positioning theory (Davies & Harré, 1990). Positions are the duties and rights that limit our choice of actions, reducing the list of what seems possible and leaving us with what is socially acceptable (Harré & Moghaddam, 2003). Davies and Harré (1990) argued that within the theory of positioning there is room to reposition oneself and others. This is a significant difference which is not afforded in ascribed roles which become fixed by services and wider social systems. Positioning then may offer us a dynamic way to begin to engage with making real social change for men and women with learning disability, for example in a university context by positioning them as: recipients of honours; expert instructors in their own lives; people who select future students; those who use the internet to find out about research; and people who belong in an academic establishment. This positions not merely the individuals themselves but invites every lecturer; student; catering assistant; vice chancellor; and other person with learning disability that they come into contact with to take on a new position in relation to the person with a learning disability. An example of this sort of positioning is seen in the work of the Teaching and Research Advisory Committee at the University of South Wales (see Hopes, 2018, for their blog).

We can also consider how to use our ability to be fluid in our own position and to not necessarily accept the positions that we are expected or asked to. For example, when in a heated debate with other professionals or relatives we could take a moment to consider the questions:

➤ *What position am I being invited into?*

➤ *How am I expected to respond here?*

➤ *In what way might I be pushing others into a particular position?*

➤ *What other positions could I take that might make something different possible?*

We can see that considering the social roles that women and men with learning disability have been allocated can help us to understand the way that meaning, language and services have been and continue to be constructed. Each context develops, and is developed by, its own discourse and results in different and often less valued outcomes for the people it was designed to serve. These meanings highlight systemic and social themes that include relationships, equality and power and it is vital that we take time to consider their impact upon what is possible when we support people living with the experience of learning disability.

References

Davies, B. & Harré, R. (1990). Positioning: The discursive production of selves. *Journal for the Theory of Social Behaviour*, 20(1), 43–63.

Duffy, S. & Perez, W. (2014). *Citizenship for All: And Accessible Guide*. Sheffield: The Centre for Welfare Reform.

Harré, R. & Moghaddam, F. (2003). Introduction: The self and others in traditional psychology and positioning theory. In R. Harré & F. Moghaddam (eds), *The Self and Others* (pp. 1–3). Westport, CT: Praeger Publishers.

Hopes, P. (2018) Teaching and Research Advisory Committee (TRAC) Blog. tracusw. blogspot.com (accessed 18 August 2018).

Stainton, T. (2008). Reason, grace and charity: Augustine and the impact of church doctrine on the construction of intellectual disability. *Disability & Society*, 23(5), 485–449.

Tuke, D. (1882). *Chapters in the History of the Insane in the British Isles*. London: Kegan Paul, Trench and Co.

Wolfensberger, W. (1972). *The Principle of Normalization in Human Services*. Toronto: National Institute on Mental Retardation.

17

Applying the Coordinated Management of Meaning in Learning Disability Services

Mark Haydon-Laurelut

> ### Accessible summary
>
> - This chapter is about communication.
>
> - Communication is what we do together.
>
> - The Coordinated Management of Meaning (CMM) is a theory that helps us to understand communication.
>
> - Communication is where people, relationships and lives are 'made'.
>
> - CMM helps us think about the kinds of stories about people and situations our communication is making.

What is the Coordinated Management of Meaning (CMM)?

CMM is a communication theory that has many connections with systemic and social constructionist ideas and practices and has been used by many systemic therapists (e.g. Cronen & Lang, 1994; Hedges, 2005; Cronen et al., 2009). CMM understands communication to be the key process through which our social worlds are made. This view is often contrasted with the transmission model of communication in which messages are passed from one (always already formed) person to another. For CMM the relational is foregrounded as the place where persons-in-conversation are made. A CMM view includes the notion that persons, their relationships, and the institutions and cultures they inhabit are made in the communication process. CMM asks us to consider the kinds of selves, relationships and social groupings that we are creating when we interact with others. It also highlights the contexts that are influencing us and those we support (the stories we have of ourselves and others) as we act into and out of the stories we carry with us. Viewing our support practices through these ideas suggests a responsibility for the co-construction ('co' because we are always involved in the social world as we do this). As we are always a part of the social world, and cannot stand outside it to comment upon it, it also suggests humility about what we can know. This has been described as participant knowledge – and opposed to spectator knowledge (Rorty, 1979 cited in Pearce, 2007). This may be an unusual idea for those trained in expert professional knowledge where a hierarchy of knowledge may be implied.

How can I put this into practice?

There are a number of CMM models that can support the use of these ideas in practice. You will find models such as the Serpentine, the Hierarchy model, Loops, and the Atomic (or Daisy) model in the CMM literature. If you want to find out more about the models, 'Using CMM' (Pearce, 1999) is a useful resource. I will introduce one model here, known as the LUUUUTT model.

Creating richer stories with the LUUUUTT model

The LUUUUTT model (see, for example, Rascon & Littlejohn, 2017) is useful in unpacking complex situations and the different ways in which they are described or 'storied'. Pearce (2007, p. 229) notes that the focus of this model is:

> on the manner of storytelling, the tension between the story told, the story lived, and/or the various 'Us'... in the situation. In my experience the client always ends up with a richer understanding of the situation than he or she had before, and is better positioned to act wisely into the situation.

For our purposes the situation may be a referral to the service in which you work, the talk that happens in a multidisciplinary team about a client and their family, a conversation(s) with a family or a text that has been written about a person such as diagnostic report, or any manner of other aspects of the working context. The LUUUUTT helps us to take a third-person position to the stories we and others are telling (Pearce, 2011, p. 27) and to ask some useful questions about what is being told and how. Let us consider the following example.

A referral is received for Nelson. It describes 'challenging behaviours' and 'autistic tendencies'. This fictional referral is written by Nelson's general practitioner (GP) following an appointment with Nelson and a member of staff from the community support team who support him for seven hours per week. The multidisciplinary team at the community learning disability service discuss the referral and place Nelson on the challenging behaviour pathway and the autism spectrum conditions diagnostic pathway. There is an initial formulation that an undiagnosed (but suspected) autism spectrum condition may be implicated in the troubling behaviour, and a wide-ranging initial assessment is booked in to ensure that Nelson's physical and mental health is thoroughly reviewed before any intervention takes place. Such an (important) assessment should support a more detailed account of the health needs of Nelson. This is, of course, particularly important given research over recent years into the marginalisation of the health needs to people with learning disability and the dire consequences. This kind of assessment is a good example of looking 'through' rather than 'at' communication, and CMM questions drawn from the LUUUUTT model may additionally sensitise us to what is being said, how it is being said and what is being made in this assessment (i.e. what the assessment is 'creating' as well as 'discovering'). For example, we may ask questions under the following headings, which fall under the LUUUUTT categories:

Stories lived

> *What are Nelson's experiences? How are these different to what is said about him?*

> *How does his best friend experience Nelson? What would he say about the issues?*

> *What are the experiences of Nelson's mother and father, of his siblings?*

> *How do support workers experience supporting Nelson?*

> *What do different system members think of what needs to happen (if anything)?*

Untold stories

> *What ideas and experiences are not discussed?*

➢ *What is known by some members of the system but not told to others (e.g. did Nelson know why he was going to see his GP)?*

➢ *What do support workers know about Nelson's past (e.g. let us say there are stories of abuse and trauma involving Nelson, known to the family and professional system but not to community support workers)?*

➢ *If stories focus on broad diagnostic or identity stories (such as the impact of autism spectrum condition or of being introverted and so on) we can zoom in and ask about the details of specific episodes of interaction and how to support better, safer, more satisfying interactions.*

➢ *If stories focus on problematic episodes we can ask: what is happening when things are going well?*

Unheard stories

➢ *If stories of deficit are dominating the referral and our assessment tools elicit only problems, how might we stay attentive to noticing stories of competence, abilities and hope?*

➢ *What does Nelson tell us (in words or by showing us with other forms of communicative action) about his experiences that are not heard?*

➢ *How is it that Nelson's repeated stories about missing his mother are not heard? Is this influenced by the weekly visits his mother makes to the house? How can we find out more about the meanings of 'missing my mum' for Nelson and for those who up to now have not 'heard' these stories?*

➢ *How might we understand Nelson differently if we listened closely to stories and actions connected to 'missing my mum'?*

Unknown stories

➢ *What do members of the current system not know about Nelson? His history? His likes? His skills?*

➢ *What do members of the system not know about each other and the current situation?*

➢ *How might understandings (stories) and actions be different if these unknown stories were known?*

Untellable stories

CMM is concerned with the logical force of an utterance – its 'oughtness'. These questions ask about what system members feel they cannot (ought not) tell:

> *What is not being said in the assessment meeting? What are the stories (e.g. of family shame concerning trans-generational mental health difficulties) that limit the contexts in which the referral might be understood?*

> *What stories are untellable in the referral (e.g. that a shortage of staff has led to Nelson being supported by an increased number of agency workers in recent months)? What would we need to do in order to support a context where this could be told?*

> *What can be told in the presence of Nelson and what cannot? What might this be making?*

> *What can we do (if we want to do anything) about this?*

Told stories

There will always be a gap between being in the world and talking about being in the world. Asking about this gap can create new understandings:

> *What conversations, between who and about what, led to the idea that the referral needed to be made?*

> *How do different members of the system (family/professionals/friends etc.) understand and talk about the issues that led to the referral?*

Story telling

> *What language is privileged and what language is marginalised? In the referral? In the multidisciplinary team meetings? In the assessment paperwork?*

> *What emotion stories are organising this work? What emotionality is shown in meetings with Nelson's family (e.g. are these meetings organised by the idea that showing emotion indicates weakness or lack of a professional or reliable storyteller)? What do shows of emotion shut down and elicit? What do we want to do about this?*

> *What impact might these kinds of storytelling have on what is known and how it is known? Does it result in diagnostic stories dominating conversations? If autism*

spectrum condition becomes the frame (the highest context) through which the issues, behaviours, relationships (the social world) is viewed, what does this obscure?

➤ *How are different kinds of storytelling coordinating (e.g. are the parents and professionals telling diagnostically influenced stories whilst Nelson and his support staff discuss episodes of difficulty in detail and with the immediate context such as place, time, mood, and relationships as the highest context)? What is the result of this lack of coordination?*

Participating in making social worlds: Concluding remarks

CMM is a large and complex theory and in this short chapter we have encountered a first taste of what it can offer. With CMM we can use any (or none) of its heuristic models and explore our work with the primary CMM questions:

'What are we making together?'
'How are we making it?'

(Pearce, 2007, p. 53)

References

Cronen, V. & Lang, P. (1994). Language and action: Wittgenstein and Dewey in the practice of therapy and consultation. *Human Systems*, 5, 5–43.

Cronen, V., Lang, P. & Lang, S. (2009). Circular questions and coordinated management of meaning theory. *Human Systems*, 20(1), 7–34.

Hedges, F. (2005). *An Introduction to Systemic Therapy with Individuals: A Social Constructionist Approach*. Basingstoke: Macmillan International Higher Education.

Pearce, W.B. (1999). Using CMM: The coordinated management of meaning. *San Mateo*. California, CA: A Pearce Associates Seminar. www.pearceassociates.com/essays/cmm_seminar.pdf (accessed 9 January 2019).

Pearce, W.B. (2007). *Making Social Worlds: A Communication Perspective*. Thousand Oaks, CA: Blackwell.

Pearce, W.B. (2011). At home in the universe with miracles and horizons: Reflections on personal and social evolution. V 3.1. www.pearceassociates.com/essays/essays_menu.htm (accessed 23 November 2017).

Rascon, N.A. & Littlejohn, S. (2017). *Coordinated Management of Meaning (CMM): A Research Manual*. Chagrin Falls, OH: Taos Institute.

18

Cultural Genograms – So Much More than a Family Tree

Jane Steeples and Abby Maitland

Accessible summary

- Genograms are a way to show someone's family tree.

- Cultural genograms can help to explore themes of identity and culture.

- A cultural genogram can support building relationships with people.

- It is important and useful to think about 'disability' on cultural genograms.

Genograms are pictorial representations of family structures (Bowen, 1978) which have been developed for clinical practice (McGoldrick et al., 2008) and used by various disciplines within the learning disabilities and non-learning disabilities fields (Pruijssers et al., 2011) for a versatile array of tasks (Barnes & Summers, 2012; van Asselt-Giverts et al., 2015). At their most basic they are an incredibly useful tool for anyone who is meeting a family for the first time and wants to begin to quickly record information in their notes about who currently lives at home, birth order, previous partners, bereavements, ages and stages of the life cycle, and the position of a person labelled with learning disability within their family. For this reason alone, being able to draw a genogram is a useful skill. However, if you draw the genogram in collaboration with an individual or family the process becomes an intervention in its own right. Through a collaborative conversation you can work together to highlight the strengths of relationships, support networks, transitions, rites of passage, family patterns and stories in the family. This can usefully invite questions about roles, expectations, similarities and possible differences in the life experiences and opportunities of the person with a learning disability and the other people in their family. Questions such as: at what age do most people in the family leave home? What does it mean to you to be an aunt or uncle? What was it like when your siblings had children? Did it make you wonder about being a parent yourself? Who supports whom? Who gets on the best? Who do you think could get on better? It is also possible to record family patterns of substance misuse, abuse and incarceration. A family genogram can open up opportunities to explore many aspects of a family's story.

Cultural genograms go a step further and specifically incorporate aspects of diversity that are pertinent to a family. This could include, but is not limited to, ethnicity, class, sexuality, disability and religion. Cultural genograms were popularised as a tool for training culturally competent family therapists by Hardy and Laszloffy (1995), who suggested that they can offer benefits in:

> ➤ Highlighting the influence of culture on a family system.

> ➤ Helping practitioners to identify their own cultural identity.

> ➤ Inviting conversations that challenge cultural assumptions and stereotypes.

> ➤ Aiding practitioners to identify their own cultural competence and learning needs.

> ➤ Helping practitioners to develop a greater awareness of how their unique cultural identities might interact with others.

Drawing a genogram

In a typical genogram you would expect to see at least three generations recorded. Usually males are signified by a square and females by a circle. For a non-binary or transgender person you should discuss with them how they would like to be recorded. Figure 18.1 shows a representation of the Simpsons' Family Genogram (with artistic licence for minor inaccuracies). You can see three generations. Homer has two half siblings from his father's previous relationships. Siblings are often recorded in age order from left to right. Marge has twin sisters, one of whom, Selma, has an adopted daughter, Ling. Marge, Homer, Bart, Lisa and Maggie all live together. The numbers in the squares and circles signify the person's age.

Pregnancies are generally recorded with a triangle and deaths with a cross through their gender symbol. However, if you are constructing the genogram with a family be sensitive to their needs and ask how they would like their bereavement to be recorded. Information about websites offering guidance

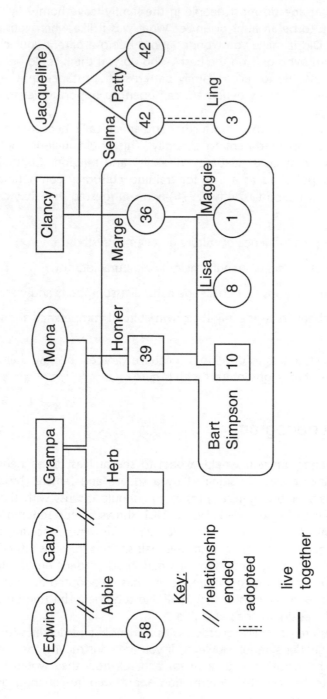

Figure 18.1 The Simpsons' Family Genogram

and software that can help with preparing genograms is included at the end of the chapter, although pen, paper and a creative imagination work just as well!

Box 18.1 A reflective exercise about your own genogram

Draw your own three-generational, cultural family tree.

- What patterns do you notice across the generations of your family?

- How might you use genograms to enhance your work with people with learning disabilities?

- Talk through your family tree with someone who you feel comfortable with. How does it feel to talk about your family? How might it feel for the people we support that we know all this about them?

Sebastian – a case study

I am a white, British, female, systemic psychotherapist, working within a multidisciplinary Child and Adolescent Mental Health Service (CAMHS) learning disability service. This case study is based on a recent piece of clinical work with Sebastian, who is 15, and his family, and illustrates how a cultural genogram was central to the work. (Sebastian is a name chosen by the client for the purpose of this book chapter and refers to his favourite TV character.)

Sebastian had a complex profile including autism, ADHD, Tourette's and moderate intellectual disability diagnoses. Sebastian displayed complex behaviours that challenged his parents and placed his two younger siblings at risk of harm. The family were Egyptian, Coptic Christians, whose first language was Arabic. They migrated to the UK when Sebastian was 12 to flee religious persecution.

When I met the family, there was a deep sense of hopelessness and despair. Sebastian's mother struggled to make sense of her son's needs and behaviours and had worries about the future implications of him 'not being normal'. She admitted to a sense of 'disconnection' from her son; this represented the loss of a former close attachment, which appeared to have been triggered by his adolescence and him beginning to challenge the family's cultural norms and values.

The challenge for me was considering how best to engage with the GRRAACCES model (Burnham, 1993) and 'working across difference': the differences between me and the family system; the differences within the family; and the differences in approach needed when working with a young person with intellectual disabilities.

Verbal approaches presented a challenge both in terms of our linguistic differences and the potential marginalisation of Sebastian from being an active participant in the therapy. Initially, Sebastian led our sessions by only engaging in playing board games together. The suggestion that we develop a cultural genogram together facilitated the movement from these initial 'play-based' sessions into something more therapeutic. It provided an essential visual tool in the work which aided and augmented verbal communication and participation.

The genogram became named 'the family map'; and was developed throughout nine months of therapeutic engagement. Sebastian engaged enthusiastically with the fabric of the 'family map' (choosing colours of pen to use, and the shapes and forms of letters and numbers) and the content (which relationship connections to focus on; family names and meanings), as well as ensuring family events, anniversaries, and especially birthdays were noted and ages changed as the weeks and months went by.

The 'family map' became collaborative and interactive. As noted by Cardone and Hilton (2006, p. 90), 'anchoring conversation in a relationship map, co-created with the person with intellectual disabilities, enhances engagement in the process.'

The 'family map' brought the family to life through the lenses of culture and religion and the use of culturally curious questions such as:

> 'Who is Sebastian most/least like in the family?'

> 'What do you think the priest would say about that issue?'

> 'What would a 16-year-old Coptic Christian boy in Egypt be doing?'

It highlighted trans-generational patterns related to expectations of marriage, heterosexuality and child-rearing; the expectations of family roles and relationships and parenting scripts; family life cycle transitions; themes of ability and disability, persecution and migration.

It created space for previously untold stories to be heard: stories of hope and resilience; re-authored stories (White & Epston, 1990) which reflected Sebastian as having competence and mastery and being the valued eldest son.

It created opportunities to reflect on key themes such as difference and similarity, ideas about normative life cycle changes and transitions, within the family's particular cultural and religious contexts (Carter & McGoldrick, 2005), and adaptation processes and changed expectations in light of having a 'different' child to any other in the family.

On reviewing the 'family map' with Sebastian and his mother they highlighted the following:-

➢ 'Learning about Mumma when she was a young girl; asking questions about her brothers and sisters.'

➢ 'Learning about family differences and similarities.'

➢ 'Celebrating Sebastian's talent of knowing all the birth dates of people in his family.'

➢ 'Talking about so many different things.'

➢ 'Mumma can know what Sebastian is thinking.'

For me, the genogram became something 'grounding', almost sacred. It brought awareness to my assumptions in a way that enhanced my cultural competence and ability to work cross-culturally in an ethical way (Britt-Krausse, 2002), deepening my regard for this family and their unique contexts.

Where's the "D" in the graces?

When training as a clinical supervisor in a predominantly systemically trained cohort, I was introduced to concepts such as Burnham's Social Graces (1993). This seemed relevant in my work as an NHS integrative counsellor with people with learning disabilities whose engagement in therapy was often aided or thwarted by their surrounding support systems. During the supervision training I noticed an emphasis on certain social graces: 'gender' and 'race' were particularly popular whilst 'ability' seemed conspicuously absent. Totsuka (2014) posed a question about which of the graces 'grab' us and which we 'distance' ourselves from. Inviting her group supervisees to enhance self-reflexivity by considering this, she found distancing to be particularly apparent with disability. Similarly, even within my experienced, culturally sensitive training cohort, 'disability' seemed marginalised. This prompted me to reflect on how wider society distances itself from people with learning disabilities, contributing to their experience of feeling unheard and voiceless (Hawkins, 2002).

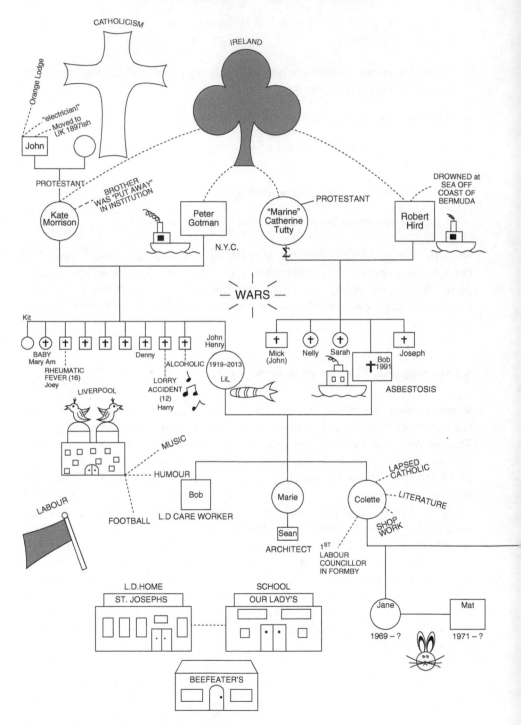

Figure 18.2   Jane's cultural genogram

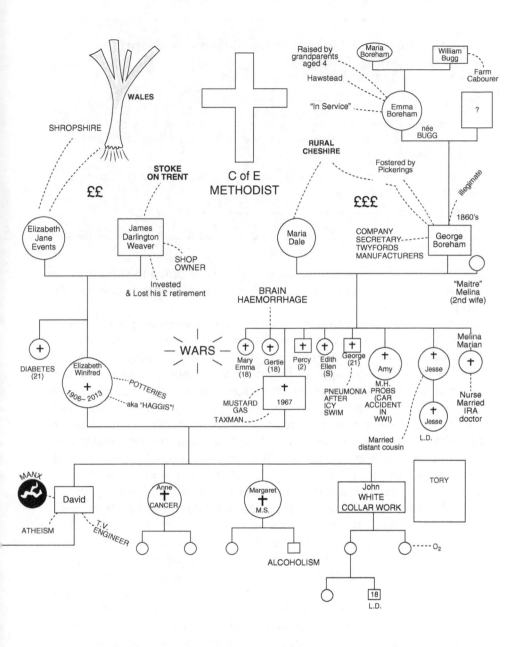

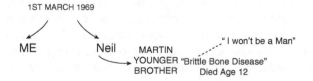

Box 18.2 Putting the lens of 'disability' onto your own
cultural genogram

Put the lens of 'disability' onto your own cultural genogram and consider the following:

● What cultural experiences have you had in your early life of 'disability'? Include
  personal experience, family, school, neighbours, TV programmes etc. Note any
  absence of experience.

● What impressions did you form about 'disability'? Think about issues of *difference*
  and how you responded to these.

● How do these experiences *help or hinder* you in your work?

As the supervisor of a group completing this activity I opted to share my own
genogram in a bid to model use of self and enhance openness within the
group (Figure 18.2).

The benefits of completing this exercise in a supervision group are wide
ranging. Supervisees who have shared their cultural genograms using the
lens of disability have commented on how the climate of safety in the group
was enhanced. They also appreciated my self-disclosures as supervisor and
how I reconnected with forgotten memories about early encounters with
'disability'. Honest reflection about ambivalent feelings when working with
'disability' and power dynamics could be tackled. It also enabled differences within the group to be explored, such as younger generations having experienced greater integration with people with disabilities at school.
Self-reflexivity was prompted, with one counsellor sharing how the exercise
enabled her to 'locate aspects of my own limitations and feelings of not
being able'. There were happy by-products too, with enhanced team cohe-
sion and appreciation of each other's rich histories and hidden diversities.
For some there were long-lasting results which enhanced practice post-
qualification. An art therapist now routinely uses genograms in her work in
higher education with students with disabilities: 'I explain what it is and in
their own time they do it and share with me if they like … after seeing students over the year we use it as a reflection piece to see what has changed.'

It is important to consider potential pitfalls when doing the exercise.
The level of personal disclosure needs to be carefully managed, especially
when working with practitioners whose training might have eschewed self-
disclosure or when there are potentially raw or shaming narratives which
people do not wish to expose at work. Participants' resistance, such as arriving late, being unprepared or forgetting to bring their genogram, needs to be
addressed sensitively. Giving express permission to have 'no go zones' during
the exercise can be beneficial.

References

Barnes, J.C. & Summers, S.J. (2012). Using systemic and psychodynamic psychotherapy with a couple in a community learning disabilities context: A case study. *British Journal of Learning Disabilities*, 40(4), 259–265.

Bowen, M. (1978). *Family Therapy In Clinical Practice*. New York: Jason Aronson.

Britt-Krausse, I. (2002). *Culture and System in Family Therapy*. London: Karnac.

Burnham, J. (1993). Systemic supervision: The evolution of reflexivity in the context of the supervisory relationship. *Human Systems*, 4, 349–381.

Cardone, D. & Hilton, A. (2006). Engaging people with intellectual disabilities in systemic therapy. In S. Baum. & H. Lynggaard. (eds), *Intellectual Disabilities – A Systemic Approach* (pp. 83–99). London: Karnac.

Carter, B. & McGoldrick, M. (2005). *The Expanded Family Life Cycle. Individual, Family and Social Perspectives*. Boston: Allyn & Bacon.

Hardy, K.V. & Laszloffy, T.A. (1995). The cultural genogram: Key to training culturally competent family therapists. *Journal of Marital and Family Therapy*, 21(3), 227–237.

Hawkins, J. (2002). *Voices of the Voiceless: Person-Centred Approaches and People with Learning Difficulties*. Ross-on-Wye: PCCS Books.

McGoldrick, M., Gerson, R. & Petry, S. (2008). *Genograms in Family Assessment* 3rd edition. New York: W.W. Norton & Co Inc.

Pruijssers, A., van Meijel, B. & van Achterberg, T. (2011). A case report for diagnosing anxiety in people with learning disabilities: The role of nurses in the application of a multidimensional diagnostic guideline. *Perspectives in Psychiatric Care*, 47(4), 204–212.

Totsuka, Y. (2014). Which aspects of the social graces grab you most? The social graces exercise for a supervision group to promote therapists' self-reflexivity. *Journal of Family Therapy*, 36(S1), 86–106.

van Asselt-Goverts, A.E., Embreghts, P.J.C.M. & Hendricks, A.H.C. (2015). Social networks of people with mild intellectual disabilities: Characteristics, satisfaction, wishes and quality of life. *Journal of Intellectual Disability Research*, 59(5), 450–461.

White, M. & Epston, D. (1990). *Narrative Means to Therapeutic Ends*. New York: Norton.

Useful websites

Genogram Analytics LLC. www.genogramanalytics.com (accessed 9 January 2019).

Gilgun, J.F. Cultural Genograms according to Hardy & Laszloffy (School of Social Work, University of Minnesota). www.slideshare.net/JaneGilgun/doing-a-cultural-genogram (accessed 9 January 2019).

19

Curiosity

Victoria Jones

Accessible summary

- It is important that we keep on finding out and trying to understand things. This is called being curious.

- It shows people that we are really interested in them.

- It makes creative ways of change possible.

- When we are not curious we can become part of the system that maintains people's problems.

- There is a Questions Card to help us be curious.

Whatever our background or goals, we work with unique human beings and our responses must necessarily be individually tailored and person-centred if they are to be effective and relationally ethical. One way to achieve this is by engaging our natural desire to explore and find out about things and apply this curiosity to the way that we connect with the human systems around us. Harnessing our own curiosity is a stance that we can take when considering a particular event, concern or relationship. It is fundamental to creating a climate where change is possible and prioritises remaining engaged with the person, their relatives, carers and colleagues whilst you explore ways of being and doing together (e.g. Cecchin, 1987; McNamee, 2005). Curiosity encourages us not to position ourselves as 'experts' and to cautiously consider the assumptions and interpretations that we make. Rather than seeking one truth, an objective answer or implying that we have an answer, a curious stance enables us to create hopeful conversations that explore possibilities, creative alternatives and change. In this way we open up infinite possibilities for collaboration and co-production.

It can be especially useful to remember to engage our curiosity when we feel that a system we are a part of has become stuck in one way of assessing, making sense, responding or intervening. For example, does your team always use the same assessment tools? If you always ask the same questions you are likely to receive the same range of answers. This might be convenient for auditing purposes but it is not going to be person-centred.

Indeed, respectful curiosity is at the heart of many of the techniques of person-centred approaches which seek to identify and create action to achieve both what is important *to* a person and what is important *for* them through coordinating the strengths, resources and knowledge of everyone in the system around them (see 'Useful Weblinks' at the end of the chapter).

Box 19.1 offers a 'Curiosity Q [Cue] Card' to help get you started.

Box 19.1 Curiosity Q Card

What other voices or views that might be influential or helpful for this person, their family or team should they/we/I consider?

Who defined the 'issue'? Who most needs change to happen?

For this issue who is/are the client/s?

In what other ways might this task be accomplished?

Am I, or others, stuck in one way of thinking about this?

In what ways and contexts might their reactions make total sense?

What might the possible consequences of this action or intervention be?

Are we using words and phrases to have the same meaning?

In what way can I be useful to you?

In what way can I make the processes of our time together more effective for us both, i.e. not just *what* we do but *how* we do it?

Taking time to consider and unpack the language we use and the sense we construct from it is also a key aspect of curiosity. If you are unsure about this idea just consider the tens, or even hundreds, of meanings that can be taken from the phrase 'I love you'. Box 19.2 gives some examples but there are many more that you can add.

> **Box 19.2 An exercise to demonstrate the relevance of exploring meaning-making in language**
>
> **'I love you' can mean...**
>
> You are nice.
>
> You are like a sister/mother/lover/uncle/grandparent to me.
>
> I want you to stop talking. Please shut up.
>
> I'm sorry.
>
> You're funny.

This highlights why it is important with that we take time to consider the way that we use language with all the people that we come into contact with as part of our work. For example, what sense are you making together of the terms: 'team'; 'family'; 'learning disability'; 'I can't cope'; and 'challenging behaviour', and what sense do you and others make of your professional role and job title?

Indeed, we can challenge ourselves to be curious about: the referral issue; possible solutions; the family concerns; the professional systems; and the processes we use, as well as our own prejudices and biases. Making our curiosity infectious and (re)awakening the curiosity of others can also be a powerful way to promote change. This requires us to practise how we make relationships with people and explore with them how we can best talk together (see Chapter 28 on relational reflexivity).

In services for people whose voice may be restricted and whose capacity may be diminished, a lack of curiosity on the part of others may be unsafe or even negligent. There are many examples of people labelled with learning disability not having their health, well-being and safeguarding needs met, arguably because no one was curious enough to find out what was going on (e.g. National Society for the Prevention of Cruelty to Children, 2003; Looking into Abuse Research Team, 2013).

Beth (not her real name) was in her late twenties when her support team observed a change in her behaviour – she had become more noisy, resistant to getting up and about, and the pace of her rocking movements had changed. She was prescribed higher levels of psychotropic medication to sedate her and manage her behaviour. Two weeks later she died from an obstructed bowel.

The assumption that it was Beth's learning disability that was the cause of the change in her behaviour was compounded by a lack of curiosity on the part of those around her about what else might be going on. These factors contributed to her death. This is an example of diagnostic overshadowing where the 'story' of learning disability overpowers our ability and willingness to ask questions that might identify physical and mental health needs (the General Medical Council has a good website on this. See 'Useful Weblinks' below). Effective, keen and thoughtful curiosity has the potential to counteract the effects of diagnostic overshadowing.

This individual lack of curiosity is also identifiable at an institutional level. All too often the deaths of people who had been labelled with a learning disability have not been systematically investigated. Just one example of this is the independent review of deaths recorded in Southern Health NHS Foundation Trust, which offered services to people with mental health needs and learning disabilities (Mazars, 2015). This reported that only 4 per cent of all 'unexpected' deaths of people labelled with learning disabilities were investigated as either a Critical Incident Review or Serious Incident Requiring Investigation (externally reportable). This compares unfavourably with reviews of 60 per cent of all 'unexpected' deaths within their Adult Mental Health Services. The Confidential Inquiry into the Premature Deaths of People with Learning Disabilities (Heslop et al., 2013) found that the most common reasons for people dying prematurely were delays and challenges in their obtaining diagnosis or treatment, and the poor provision of appropriate care when their needs changed. When that happens, a lack of curiosity on the part of services and organisations prevents us from learning how to avoid repeating our death-making mistakes in the future. Our institutional lack of curiosity leaves women and men with learning disabilities more vulnerable to an early death.

We can use curiosity to engage ourselves and others in creating relationships, maintaining conversations and exploring possibilities for change together. Curiosity can show people that we are really interested in them and what they have to say. It can help us consider *how* we do things as well as *what* it is that we do. Ultimately, when we support people labelled with learning disabilities, increasing our curiosity can also enhance our potential to promote a good life, improve safeguarding and save lives.

References

Cecchin, G. (1987). Hypothesizing-circularity-neutrality revisited: An invitation to curiosity. *Family Process*, 26, 405–413.

Heslop, P., Blair, P., Fleming, P., Hoghton, M., Marriott, A. & Russ, L. (2013). *Confidential Inquiry into Premature Deaths of People with Learning Disabilities (CIPOLD): Final Report*. Bristol: Norah Fry Research Centre.

Looking into Abuse Research Team (2013). *Looking into Abuse: Research by People with Learning Disabilities*. Pontypridd, Wales: University of Glamorgan, Rhondda

Cynon Taff People First and New Pathways udid.research.southwales.ac.uk/
media/files/documents/2013-03-05/Final_report.pdf (accessed 28 February
2018).

Mazars (2015). *Independent Review of Deaths of People with a Learning Disability
or Mental Health Problem in Contact with Southern Health NHS Foundation Trust
April 2011 to March 2015*. London: Mazars.

McNamee, S., 2005. Curiosity and irreverence: Constructing therapeutic
possibilities. *Human Systems* 16, 75–84.

National Society for the Prevention of Cruelty to Children (2003). *It Doesn't Happen
to Disabled Children': Child Protection and Disabled Children*. London: NSPCC.

Useful Weblinks

General Medical Council (2018). *Discrimination*. www.gmc-uk.org/
learningdisabilities/200.aspx (accessed 1 April 2018).

Helen Sanderson Associates (undated). *Home Page*. www.helensandersonassociates.
co.uk (accessed 28 February 2018).

Looking into Abuse: research by people with learning disabilities http://udid.
research.southwales.ac.uk/trac/research/trac/lia/ (accessed 25 February 2019).
Make sure that you look at the accessible literature review section.

20

Diversity IS GRACE – Using the 'Social Graces' to Promote Reflection on Diversity

Victoria Jones

Accessible summary

- It is important to recognise and respect people's differences.

- The 'social graces' can help us to remember some of the ways that people are different.

- You cannot always see people's differences.

- We need to think about why we talk about some differences more than others.

- Intersectionality says that we should not think about one difference at a time.

- We all have more than one difference happening at the same time and together they make a whole new way of being different.

- 'Diversity IS GRACE' can help us remember all of these things.

Whatever professional hat you wear (or are hoping to wear), your regulating body will require you to comply with equality and diversity policies and legislation. However, ethical and effective practice regarding diversity in a helping relationship arises not from observing guidance but through a significant degree of reflective and reflexive practice. The 'social graces' is a mnemonic tool developed by Burnham and Roper-Hall to help us consider our practice in relation to aspects of diversity and difference (Burnham, 2012). Burnham describes how he wanted to aid his students to remember more aspects of difference and societal prejudice, qualities that might attract an 'ism' and therefore require aware attention, by offering them the acronym as a prompt. These differences are performed and constructed in *social* settings although we can also consider the *personal* aspects of how they are experienced and the recursive (interwoven and constantly reiterating) relationship between these two aspects (Burnham, 2012); for an example refer to Chapter 3 in this text. In its most simplistic form the idea of the 'social graces' reminds us to consider aspects of our own and our clients' legally protected characteristics under the Equality Act (2010), i.e. race (including colour, nationality, ethnic or national origin), religion (or lack of it), age, ability, expectant or on maternity leave, sexual orientation, sex and being or becoming a transsexual person. These represent traits that are currently recognised in law largely because they are considered immutable (outside of the control of the person themselves).

However, the 'social graces' concept was always more inclusive. Gender; geography; appearance; class; culture; education; economics; employment and spirituality were also identified as 'social graces' early in the development of the tool. This was never intended as a finite list. The invitation exists for us to consider what other social graces can be added that have meaning and significance to us, our clients and our work together. These are factors that may have an impact upon both how we experience and are experienced by each other (Burnham, 2012). It is also important to consider in what ways our social graces might interact with those of other people (Burnham & Roper-Hall, 2017). These are critical considerations in a systemic approach to diversity that have the potential to facilitate and catalyse our critical and reflexive thinking about diversity in every area of our practice.

Like all tools that offer to reduce a complex and important issue into something that can be easily remembered, the 'social graces' is at risk of being used to over-simplify things. Some questions that arise from such an aide-memoire include: who says what can (or should) be included in the expanded list? Who are we as systemic thinkers to be in charge of the list? In what way does the list open up my thinking about aspects of diversity and what might it be closing down? (Mills, 2017). For example, it is possible to add 'accent' because there is an 'a' in graces, and this characteristic might have a huge impact on social relationships, identity, standing, access to resources and the impression made on others. A person's speech may be perfectly understandable by their family but virtually unintelligible to the people who support them at a day centre, which might afford them a different but relationally meaningful experience in each context. But what about our differences that do not begin with those six letters: F for feminist, I for impairment or D for disabled to give just three examples (Jones & Reeve, 2014, 2017)?

> ### Box 20.1 Using curiosity around aspects of diversity
>
> What aspects of your own difference are important to you but not covered by the letters G, R, A, C, E and S?
>
> What are you curious about when asked to think about someone's ethnicity or culture?
>
> Are you equally curious when asked to consider impairment, ability or disability?

Burnham usefully distinguishes between social graces that are visible or invisible and voiced or unvoiced. The former explores how readily a person's social graces can be identified by or shown to others, for example a person who uses a wheelchair due to a physical impairment as opposed to someone with a learning disability who has no mobility issues. Both people experience living with impairment and may feel the effects of psycho-emotional disablism (see Chapter 3), yet for one of these people their particular aspect of diversity may not be immediately apparent. From a systemic point of view this will have an impact upon both how we enter into and how we make sense of being with clients, families, colleagues and other professionals. Our relationships with our own social graces can affect whether we want them to be visible or not and to what extent we choose to show them. Of course, it is also true that the relationship that other people have with our differences may also impact upon how much we feel we are willing or able to show them. This invites us to consider: what aspects of our own social graces do we show to others without necessarily even thinking about it? For example, I have an English accent, Irish ancestry, celebrate living in Wales, sport a rainbow lanyard, have pale skin, wear a ring on my wedding finger and jeans to work, have greying 80s-style curly hair, the Guardian app on my Apple phone, and audibly creaky knees. What would you take from me about my visible social graces and in what ways might they collide with your own social graces, whether they are visible or not?

'Voiced or unvoiced' invites us to consider whether and how aspects of diversity are alluded to by the person/family themselves or the practitioner. This is not as simple as it might sound as our own prejudices, beliefs and knowledge will all come into play. Something might not be spoken about or referred to for a wide range of reasons and often for more than one reason at the same time. Burnham suggested social graces might go unvoiced because of:

> being outside awareness; seeing but not noticing; perception of relevance; not realising the significance; taken for granted; cultural rules of politeness; not having

words to name/describe, or not having a culturally appropriate question/grammar; waiting for someone else to say something; or if the practitioner does not mention it then it cannot be important.

(2012, p. 147)

A key challenge is to notice in our practice when we see patterns of privileging, or voicing, certain graces over others (which we may even leave unvoiced). We can use reflective practice, reflexivity and supervision to consider what skills, knowledge and experience we might need to develop in order to be able to begin to cautiously and sensitively explore with our clients the social graces that are important and useful to them and our work together.

Box 20.2 An exercise to explore how we 'notice' diversity

Figure 20.1 highlights how easy it is for some 'social graces' to be more visible than others. Look at the diagram for up to 10 seconds and ask a colleague to do the same. Stop looking at the diagram and discuss the words that you remember jumping out at you. Consider: what is it about my background; vocabulary; experience and knowledge that may have led to me seeing the 'social graces' that I did? Which ones are there that I did not even notice? Whilst this might reflect your eyesight as much as your awareness of 'social graces', it offers an interesting metaphor for what can happen when we meet and work with people.

Think of people that you have supported – which of their social graces were visible/invisible and voiced/unvoiced?

To what extent do we and our services 'privilege' learning disability over a person's other diverse identities?

In what ways do you and your colleagues support people to experience their diverse identities?

Intersectionality

It is critical that we do not think of diversity as simply a list of characteristics, despite the possible invitation of the Equality Act and the 'social graces' to do so. Intersectionality is a theory that recognises that oppressions do not operate in isolation and are interconnected (Hill, Collins & Bilge, 2016). It challenges us not to think of distinct categories of difference but to recognise that they do not accumulate or multiply in effect but rather create individual lived experience. Consider Li Na, a woman of Chinese heritage who has been labelled with a learning disability and identifies as lesbian. She will have a

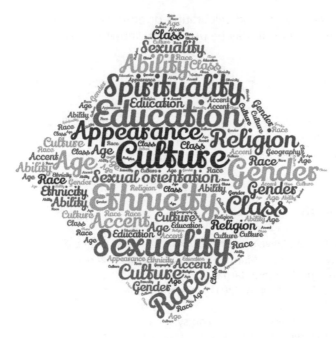

Figure 20.1   A word cloud of the 'social graces', similar to Burnham's collide-scope (2012)

unique perspective and understanding of what it means to be her. Li Na, like all of us, 'will always be made up of the overlap, or intersections, of [these] different aspects of identity, which are bound within contexts of power that give them meaning' (Butler, 2017, p. 16). Intersectionality reminds us that we are each more than the sum of our parts. In the same way that I could not take a carrot cake and return it to eggs, flour, sugar, butter and carrots, I am unable to separate out the constituent parts of my own social graces. Nor can I make sense of me and my life experiences in terms of single parts of myself. The way that our personal and social graces have been processed together through time, contexts, relationships, language and storying make us the unique individuals that we are.

We are legally, professionally and ethically obliged to consider aspects of equality and diversity in our practice. This necessarily entails considering our own characteristics of difference and how they may interact with those of the people we support and work with. Our identities are formed through an inter-woven and interconnected union of all our 'social graces' and those of the people around us. Reflection, reflexive practice and supervision offer us keys to working effectively with all aspects of diversity.

The word 'grace' has many meanings: polite and decent behaviour, an admirable quality, a capacity to accommodate, and beauty. It is probably fair to say that recognising and celebrating diversity can help us to achieve these things in our practice. It may be useful to acknowledge and remember that

Diversity IS GRACE.

In this way we are usefully reminded to consider Disability, Impairment and InterSectionality (IS) whilst emphasising the importance of diversity whatever letter our differences happen to start with.

References

Burnham, J. (2012). Developments in social GRRRAAACCEEESSS: visible-invisible and voiced-unvoiced, *Mutual Perspectives culture and reflexivity in systemic psychotherapy*. London: Karnac Books Ltd.

Burnham, J. & Roper-Hall, A. (2017). Commentaries on this issue. *Context*, 151(June), 47–50.

Butler, C. (2017). Intersectionality and systemic therapy. *Context*, 151(June), 16–18.

Hill Collins, P. & Bilge, S. (2016). *Intersectionality*. Cambridge: Polity Press.

Jones, V. & Reeve, D. (2014). *DISsing the Social GGRRAAACCEEESSS*. Presentation to the Association for Family Therapy Conference in Liverpool, 20 September 2014.

Jones, V. & Reeve, D. (2017). 'Dissing' the social graces. *Context*, 151, June, 38–40.

Legislation.gov.uk. (2010). *Equality Act 2010*. www.legislation.gov.uk/ukpga/2010/15/contents (accessed 25 February 2018).

Mills, S. (2017). Be-wilder. *Context*, 151, June, 34–37.

21

Engaging People with Learning Disabilities in Family and Network Meetings

Sandra Baum and Julie Steel

Accessible summary

- All people with learning disabilities should be asked to come to meetings about themselves.

- It is important to think about the best ways to help people take part in meetings.

- Planning before meetings is important.

- There are ways to include the voice of people who don't use words.

In learning disabilities services we work with a range of people with mild to profound learning disabilities. In order to decide whether we conduct a family therapy session or a network meeting, we consider the following questions: Who wants what for whom? Who needs to be in conversation with whom, and about what (Lang & McAdam, 1995)? Who needs to change (Rikberg Smyly, 2006)? Whichever meeting is arranged, we always ask the person with learning disabilities to attend and this is not dependent on their communication skills or level of ability. This chapter summarises how we prepare the sessions, how we engage people with learning disabilities in sessions, and how we include the voice of a person without words (a person with no verbal communication) by 'stepping into the shoes of the other' (Iveson, 1990, pp. 82–83).

Preparing for family sessions and network meetings

We are always mindful of the importance of 'well begun is half done' (Lang & McAdam, 1995, p. 78) and thus we take time to prepare the sessions before they take place by considering how to set up the room, for example position- ing the seats so that everyone can see each other. We consider how we can create a context so that all involved can feel respected, heard, listened to and included (Anderson & Johnson, 2010). We therefore greet the person with learning disabilities and their family in the waiting room and first invite the person with learning disabilities into the session and ask where they would like to sit and where they would like others to sit (Fredman, 2014). We begin by explaining who we are and that we are here to offer different ideas. In the session we seek permission from everyone about what is acceptable to talk about and what is off limits (see Fredman, 2014). We are mindful of how we enable the person with learning disabilities to feel that they are central to the conversation and we do this by using pens and a large sheet of paper to write down key words or phrases about what they and everyone would like to talk about (Fredman & Lynggaard, 2015). Also to enable participation, we tune in to non-verbal expressions or a change of voice, tone or pitch, intonation or body posture, which may accompany key words or phrases spoken by the person with learning disabilities as 'they seem to call for a response and they touch or move the speaker and/or the listener' (Fredman & Lynggaard, 2015, p. 23). We always use simple language; paraphrase what has been said; slow down the pace; and summarise conversations at appropriate intervals. We take care to check our understanding of words that everyone uses so that we do not impose our meanings on them (Lynggaard & Baum, 2006). We some- times 'lend the words' to people with learning disabilities (Booth & Booth, 1996) by trying out different but similar words that might fit for them.

Other ideas that we have found useful to support understanding and develop a shared language include:

> Using gestures to accompany speech, for example using a 'thumbs up' sign to check out whether the person is happy to talk about a particular issue.

> Using 'externalisation' (White & Epston, 1990) in order to view the prob- lem as outside the person. Ways to separate problems from people include objectifying feelings (e.g. 'the anxiety', 'the guilt'); asking people to think of the problem as being a 'thing' (Morgan, 2000); asking people to draw what they think the problem looks like; and asking people to give the problem a name to personify it (e.g. naming anger as 'Mr Shouty'). Such techniques can help make these abstract concepts more concrete for the person with learning disabilities (see McFarlane & Lynggaard, 2009).

➤ Using the characters from TV programmes such as BBC1's *EastEnders* that are familiar to people with learning disabilities to help them to open up conversations about life events that they might find difficult to explain (Cardone & Hilton, 2006); for example discussing family relationships by asking 'which character each family member thought he or she was and the meaning of this' (Cardone & Hilton, 2006, p. 94).

➤ Using visual images to describe the impact of events or experiences on the person with learning disabilities (Baum, 2017). For example, 'If you were to paint a picture [of what we have talked about] what would it look like?' (Baum, 2017, p. 49) Such questions can help people with learning disabilities to participate in the session in a fun way and they often relate to images better than the spoken word (Baum, 2017).

Including the voice of a person without words/no verbal communication

We are mindful of how a person with profound learning disabilities can participate in the session. Additional preparations may be necessary to support their inclusion. We have found the questions outlined by Lynggaard (2012) very useful in considering how to maximise inclusivity:

➤ How might we arrange our seating so the person feels comfortable?

➤ Who knows them best?

➤ What might they like or need to feel comfortable?

➤ Who would they like to keep within eyesight?

➤ How can we best prepare our emotional postures? (Lynggaard, 2012, p. 13).

During the session, the perspective of the person without a speaking voice can be brought into the room through the questions we ask of those who are significant in their life. An example of this is inviting another person to speak from two positions: their own position and the position of the person without words (Iveson, 1990). The therapist asks others in the meeting who would be prepared to speak twice, once for themselves and once for the person without a speaking voice. Care is taken to highlight that the purpose of the task is to invite the client's perspective and not to be concerned about 'getting it right'. Some people may find it hard to speak from the position of someone else. We thus ask questions like 'I wonder what the world might look like through their eyes, and how they experience their surroundings and us?' (Lynggaard, 2012, p. 15)

We ask about what others think the person without a speaking voice might be communicating with their behaviour. In addition, the therapist may tentatively hypothesise what the person may be experiencing, 'in the hope of finding something that fits and enables us to anchor meaning for a while, and thereby know how to go on' (Lynggaard, 2012, p. 16). We, therefore, invite people to 'step into the shoes of the other' by reflecting on the client's position and experiences.

Conclusion

On the surface, engaging with people with learning disabilities in systemic practice can be challenging; however, by adapting techniques which are outlined in this chapter it is possible to make the process much more inclusive, and one that values the person at the centre of the work.

References

Anderson, E. & Johnson, S. (2010). Older people and their significant systems: Meeting with families and networks. In G. Fredman, E. Anderson & J. Stott (eds), *Being with Older People: A Systemic Approach* (pp. 113–139). London: Karnac Books.

Baum, S. (2017). How to end therapeutic work with people with learning disabilities using outsider witnessing practices. *The Bulletin of the Faculty for People with Intellectual Disabilities*, 15(3) Dec, 45–51.

Booth, T. & Booth, W. (1996). Sounds of silence: Narrative research with inarticulate subjects. *Disability and Society*, 11(1), 55–69.

Cardone, D. & Hilton, A. (2006). Engaging people with intellectual disabilities in systemic therapy. In S. Baum & H. Lynggaard (eds), *Intellectual Disabilities: A Systemic Approach* (pp. 83–99). London: Karnac Books.

Fredman, G. (2014). Weaving net-works of hope with families, practitioners and communities: Inspirations from systemic and narrative approaches. *Australian and New Zealand Journal of Family Therapy*, 35, 54–71.

Fredman, G. & Lynggaard, H. (2015). Braiding hopes and intentions with people affected by intellectual disabilities, and their networks of family and carers. *Context*, 138, 22–26.

Iveson, C. (1990). *Whose Life? Community Care of Older People and Their Families*. London: BT Press.

Lang, P. & McAdam, E. (1995). Stories, giving accounts and systemic descriptions. Perspectives and positions in conversations. Feeding and fanning the winds of creative imagination. *Human Systems: The Journal of Systemic Consultation and Management*, 6, 71–103.

Lynggaard, H. (2012). Something understood – Something misunderstood. *Clinical Psychology and People with Learning Disabilities*, 10(2), 12–18.

Lynggaard, H. & Baum, S. (2006). So how do I…? In S. Baum & H. Lynggaard (eds), *Intellectual Disabilities: A Systemic Approach* (pp. 185–202). London: Karnac Books.

McFarlane, F. & Lynggaard, H. (2009). The taming of Ferdinand: Narrative therapy and people affected with intellectual disabilities. *The International Journal of Narrative Therapy and Community Work*, 3, 19–26.

Morgan, A. (2000). *What is Narrative Therapy?* Adelaide: Dulwich Centre Publications.

Rikberg Smyly, S. (2006). Who needs to change? Using systemic ideas when working in group homes. In S. Baum & H. Lynggaard (eds), *Intellectual Disabilities: A Systemic Approach* (pp. 142–163). London: Karnac Books.

White, M. & Epston, D. (1990). *Narrative Means to Therapeutic Ends*. New York: W.W. Norton.

22

From Either/Or to Both/And

Victoria Jones and Mark Haydon-Laurelut

Accessible summary

- It can be helpful to think that things can be more than one thing at the same time.

- The picture on the next page shows this: it is *both* an old woman *and* a young woman.

- This can be an especially helpful way to look at things when people feel stuck and are not sure about how to move forwards.

- But it can make things feel less certain and less safe, too, so it is important to support people well when we help them to think this way.

Q: What is the difference between an optimist and a pessimist?

A: The optimist thinks that this is the best of all possible worlds,
      The pessimist fears the optimist may be right!

Most of us like to be right. There is a human tendency to try and simplify things, look for certainties and avoid doubt. When we think that there is only one truth, or a simpler way of seeing and doing things, we are being *reductionist*. The quest for best outcomes informed by evidence-based practice is arguably based on this premise. However, a systemic and constructionist perspective acknowledges that there are multiple realities that simultaneously coexist. This means that there are also multiple truths. Consider Figure 22.1, which contains both a beautiful young woman and an older woman with a big nose. We are often drawn towards seeing one or the other of the available images or possibilities when it is the case that they coexist simultaneously. The

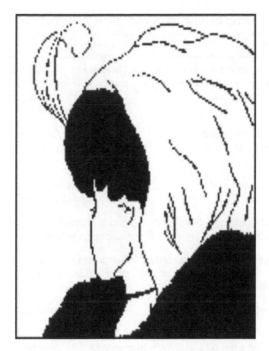

Figure 22.1   Showing *both* an old woman *and* a young woman coexisting simultaneously

(Hill, 1915)

image is not more one woman than the other and there is no 'right way' or 'wrong way' to see the picture.

It has been found that supporting people to consider moving from an either/or position to a recognition of both/and can be useful in helping them to bring about change (Andersen, 1987). An example of this could be seen in working with a struggling mum. She and those around her may be caught in the question of whether she is a good mother or a bad mother. This asks her to take a position that is either 'off the hook' (she is good, her work is done) or 'shamed' (she is not fit to be a mother and her children do not deserve her). Neither of these views will be likely to enable her to engage with you in making change to be the best mum that she can be. However, it is also possible to consider that she is *both* the best mother her children have ever had *and* the worst mother they have ever had. Supporting her to recognise both these realities can help you to create a relationship that enables you both to celebrate what is going well and explore what might be able to go better. Of course, this is true for all parents and so the both/and technique can also help you to draw commonalities with the experiences of others. Table 22.1 gives

Table 22.1　Illustrating examples of moving from either/or to both/and

From either/or...	To both/and...
Either 'A person's diagnosis is responsible for their behaviour,' or 'The person is responsible for their behaviour'.	There are many contexts, including a particular diagnosis and the person's unique identity, that contribute to the person's behaviour.
Either 'The person is the problem,' or 'The carer/relative is the problem'.	Maybe the person and the relative/carer are both part of the problem and part of the solution.
'Either she is losing it or I am.'	Or possibly you both are losing it and totally sane all at once?
Either 'She has the mental age of a 7 year old' or 'She is a grown woman'.	She is a grown woman who also needs support to understand.
Either 'Being the parent of a disabled child is bloody hard,' or 'Being the parent of a disabled child is utterly amazing'.	Being the parent of a disabled child can be both bloody hard and utterly amazing.
In this situation am I a practitioner or a researcher?	I am both a practitioner and a researcher.
What examples can you add from your own experiences?	

examples of the either/or thinking that can go on in services for people with learning disabilities and offers examples of both/and alternatives.

Both/and can be a useful way to acknowledge and begin to work with complexity in the systems that we support and are part of. It gives us permission to feel confused or overwhelmed and to hold, without necessarily being able to resolve, apparent contradictions, risk and complexity. The opportunity to encounter more than one truth through viewing situations, problems or referrals through multiple contexts (of time, theory, emotion, person or perspective, for example) can enable us to avoid seeking a single solution.

Considering both/and can help us to introduce tentative questions about alternative possibilities – what makes it hard to see the other way? What might it mean to you if they are both 'true'? This can be a helpful way to see alternatives when people (individuals, families, carers and teams) have become stuck. Mason considered that we need to be able to tolerate uncertainty and doubt before we can take on board new ideas (1993). He proposed a grid that can help us think about people's readiness for change (our own and others'). There are two axes, one from unsafe to safe and the other from certain to uncertain. Mason's grid is reproduced in Figure 22.2.

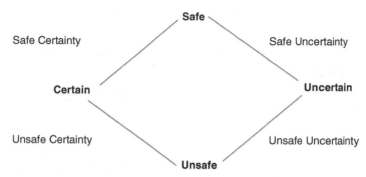

Figure 22.2   Mason's factors influencing readiness to change and consider new ideas (Mason, 1993, p.195)

Moving towards safe uncertainty

To facilitate change and development our task is to support ourselves and others to move towards positions where we can feel both safe and uncertain. In other words, we need to create a context in which we feel safe enough to feel uncertain and to live with not-knowing. Using the both/and technique can be useful to create a context where this is possible.

References

Andersen, T. (1987). The reflecting team: dialogue and meta-dialogue in clinical work. *Family Process, 26,* 415–428.

Hill, W.E. (1915). My wife and my mother-in-law. *Puck,* 16(11), Nov.

Mason, B. (1993). Towards positions of safe uncertainty. *Human Systems: The Journal of Systemic Consultation and Management, 4,* 189–200.

23

Irreverence

Victoria Jones

Accessible summary

- We need to not get stuck doing things in only one way.
- Being irreverent means asking questions and having ideas.
- Being irreverent is about trying different ways of doing things.
- Not being sure about something (doubt) can be really useful.

When you have spent time, energy and sometimes even tears in your quest to become a professional who works with and for people with learning disabilities, their families and systems, it is easy to become attached to the theories that you have put so much effort into studying. It is also often helpful to you as an employee and colleague to have faith that the systems, processes and services that you work with and for actually achieve the effective, individualised and specific services that they purport to offer people (in 1975 Wolfensberger and Glenn called this *model coherency*). It is easy to become emotionally and intellectually attached to the ideas, culture and profession that you have worked so long and hard to belong to. Cecchin et al. (1992) considered that this situation creates a potential hazard for good practice. They suggest that having too much reliance on, or belief in, a particular approach, culture or way of doing things can risk us becoming inflexible in a way that is detrimental to the quality and outcomes of the service we offer.

For example, you get a new job in a service supporting people with learning disabilities and after a few weeks of taking it all in you have an idea that you think might be useful to help a client cope better with an activity. Your idea involves a new way of doing something but when you propose it in a team meeting, two staff clearly state that 'it will not work' and 'something similar was tried before'. These experienced staff are relying on the way that they have become accustomed to working, are resistant to trying something new, and appear unwilling to entertain a new idea that may be in the best interests of their client. This could raise a question regarding whether their practice is person centred or ethical, or it may simply be that they disagree with you. Equally, if your new idea is the current evidence-based trend or something you have successfully offered to a number of clients previously and you have not taken a moment to consider whether this is the right thing, at the right time, for this person, in this context, then it is possible that your practice may be as poor as your colleagues'.

Cecchin et al. (1992) proposed that we need to learn to be *irreverent* towards our ideas. Doubt is the basis of irreverence. We need to learn to notice when we are uncomfortable with the way things are and develop questions about what is happening. In this way we can begin to celebrate uncertainty and make it useful to ourselves, our practice and the people that we support. Irreverence is an ability to be comfortable with doubt and live with uncertainty, to ask questions and not grow weary. It can be difficult to hold a position of doubt when we are constantly pushed towards practice that is based in the best evidence, thus making it the closest we can get to a certainty that we have 'done the right thing'. Key to effective irreverence and model coherency is truly person-centred practice, even when that goes against the latest research.

This is not to say that all theories and concepts are inherently useless and there is no point studying them (if that was the case we would not have written this book). Cecchin et al. (1992) also emphasised that in order to be truly irreverent to a concept it is important to be sure that you know it well. This increases the chance that you will not 'throw the baby out with the bathwater' (or get rid of what is working well in an effort to dispose of what is not working well) and also ensures that you know the basic ethical and professional concepts.

Irreverence is about being prepared to accept the role of devil's advocate, to put ideas out there whilst being brave enough to say something new, different or controversial, *but at the same time* not being convinced that your idea is the true or only way. It is about making suggestions rather than finding solutions. Irreverence is about advocating that everyone in a service system remains open to considering different ideas. As a consequence, irreverence is also a crucial factor in enabling staff to raise concerns. If we are not wedded to one particular way of doing something, or beholden to the service system and its ways of working, it is easier to continue to be curious about it. To be an irreverent practitioner means to be effective at asking awkward or challenging questions and not accepting poor practice. Arguably, whistle-blowers embody irreverence to the system that employs them and the poor practice that concerns them. This suggests that in order to be an ethical professional we require a degree of commitment to irreverence. Cecchin et al. (1992) acknowledged that it can take courage to question what it is that you think you know about something and about what is working, and to take action in a direction that you may not be accustomed to or as familiar with.

Indeed, Duncan et al. (2015) considered that *constructive dissent,* sharing different ideas from the rest of the team in the interests of better outcomes for clients, can be useful to enhance decision making, problem solving, new ideas and improved group outcomes. They proposed that team leaders and managers should seek to create a work culture where it is encouraged and accepted that team members will offer different ideas and that doing so is in the best interests of everyone. In such teams there would be: a willingness to live with uncertainty; no such thing as a bad idea; and nothing that could not be changed if it became less effective or useful to the person being supported.

Coming up with new ideas that may or may not be useful is the heart of change – both in the moments we share with the people we meet day to day and in creating the sparks that initiate wider campaigns and movements. However, it is important to avoid the trap of thinking that being a campaigner is the same thing as being irreverent. By necessity a campaigner needs to be passionately enthusiastic and committed to the idea that they are seeking to promote. To be really irreverent you need to be as ready to jettison your new idea as you are to make a change in the existing theories, models, hypotheses and formulations that influence your work. Campaigns have made a significant difference to our communities and the lived experience of people with learning disability. For example, the Paul Ridd Foundation has made a huge impact on standards for hospital care for people with learning disabilities living in Wales; the Justice for LB campaign led by the Ryan family highlighted poor care standards in England; Be the Change is a Scottish campaign against bullying of people with learning disabilities; and Inclusion Ireland seeks fully accessible changing places that promote people's rights not to be treated in inhuman and degrading ways. These campaigns are developed by people who have a specific goal of large-scale social change in mind. They are on a mission that requires decisiveness and purpose and has very little room for doubt, and is thus incompatible with irreverence. However, whilst the campaign trail itself is almost the antithesis of irreverence the journey to that trail is often established through it. If the Ridd and Ryan families had not held doubt about the way their relatives died; if people in Scotland had accepted that so many people with learning disabilities were at risk of being bullied; or if, in Ireland, they had not thought that dignity was a basic human right for all, these campaigns for wider social change would never have started.

Irreverence has relevance to both individual professionals and teams. We all need to find ways to embrace doubt and to practise making it useful to achieve better outcomes for the people we support. In doing so we offer ourselves an opportunity to hold onto hope and to sustain the enthusiasm and passion that first brought us into supporting people with learning disabilities.

References

Cecchin, G., Lane, G. & Ray, W. (1992). *Irreverence: A Strategy for Therapists' Survival.* London: Karnac.

Duncan, J., Waytz, A. & Young, L. (2015). The psychology of whistleblowing. *Current Opinion in Psychology, 6,* 129–133.

Wolfensberger, W. & Glenn, L. (1975). *Program Analysis of Service Systems (PASS): A Method for the Quantitative Evaluation of Human Services. Vol. 1. Handbook.* 3rd ed. Toronto: National Institute on Mental Retardation.

Campaign Links

Enable Scotland, Be the Change campaign. www.enable.org.uk/change-get-know/.

Justice for LB campaign. www.justiceforlb.org.

Paul Ridd Foundation. www.paulriddfoundation.org.

Changing Places Ireland campaign. www.inclusionireland.ie.

24

My Restraint Story: A Communication Tool to Facilitate A Conversation following the Use of Restrictive Interventions

Samuel Coe

Accessible summary

- Experiencing physical restraint can be extremely difficult for people.

- After someone has been restrained or seen a restraint they should have a chance to talk about it. This is called a debrief.

- Debriefs using pictures as well as words may be useful for people with a learning disability.

- This chapter talks about two debrief tools which use pictures to help make sense of what happened.

- One is for someone who has been restrained and the other is for someone who saw someone else be restrained.

- The tools have been reviewed by people with learning disability.

Following the Winterbourne scandal (Department of Health, 2012), there is a national drive to reduce restrictive interventions (Department of Health, 2015) that are used on people with learning disability. The Department of Health (2014) described in their *Positive and Proactive Care* guidance that a restrictive intervention is: 'The deliberate acts on the part of other person(s) that restrict an individual's movement, liberty and/or freedom to act independently'. This can include physical restraint, mechanical restraint (use of equipment and devices), chemical restraint (use of medication), seclusion or long-term segregation. Restrictive interventions can be used if there is a real possibility of harm to the person, staff or the public if no action is undertaken;

any restraint should not be done for longer than absolutely necessary and only ever used as a last resort (Department of Health, 2014). The nature of techniques used must also be proportionate to the risk of harm, and professional carers supporting people with learning disabilities should seek to maintain the dignity of the person and eliminate painful restraint (Department of Health, 2014).

I work at an inpatient Assessment and Treatment Unit (ATU) for people with learning disability where a restraint reduction programme (toolkit) has been implemented. One aspect of the toolkit is a quarterly audit, which looks for trends and patterns in restrictive interventions and facilitates consideration of how we can promote proactive strategies so that restraint is used as little as possible. The number of restraints used and the use of more restrictive restraint techniques (such as prone, when a person is held on the floor face down) have shown a decrease since recordings began.

NICE Guidelines (2015) suggest that a person who has been restrained should be involved in an immediate individual debrief and that this should take place as soon as possible after they have recovered their composure. The quarterly audits in our ATU indicated that debriefs were being routinely offered to clients after incidents; however, this was done in a verbal way. The NICE guidance (2015) sets out some standards about what should be covered in an immediate debrief, which aims to:

➤ Acknowledge the emotional responses to the incident and assess whether there is a need for emotional support for any trauma experienced.

➤ Determine the factors that contributed to an incident that led to a restrictive intervention, identify any factors that can be addressed quickly to reduce the likelihood of a further incident, and amend risk and care plans accordingly.

➤ Promote relaxation and feelings of safety, and support a return to normal patterns of activity.

➤ Ensure that everyone involved in the client's care has been informed of the event, if the service user agrees.

However, this guidance does not acknowledge the reasonable adjustments needed to make it accessible, useful and person-centred for people with learning disability. All too often, the voice of the person who is restrained is left out. Making the debrief processes accessible may help to make this voice heard.

Another part of the restraint reduction toolkit at the ATU is the client perspective audit. This looks into the client's attitudes and experience of restrictive interventions and, unsurprisingly, clients have told us that being restrained can be really difficult. With support and through conversation, the team and clients concluded that if people do not understand why they were restrained (or why other clients were), it can make it even more difficult to experience or observe. Few studies have looked at people's experience *during* physical restraint, but findings suggest people can feel distressed and ignored *prior to* the use of restraint (Bonner et al., 2002), and angered and panicked (Sequeira & Halstead, 2002) or isolated and ashamed (Bonner et al., 2002) *following* the use of restrictive interventions. These findings of heavily emotion-laden responses suggest that a predominantly verbal approach to debrief might be difficult for anyone. Debriefing after restraint is clearly important to reduce distress and support a return to individual and ward 'equilibrium' and to provide a feedback loop through more formal review processes (Sutton et al., 2014), but it can be difficult for people to talk about what happened. These difficulties can be exacerbated for people who experience communication difficulties, particularly when they are in a new communication environment such as the ATU.

To address this, a user-friendly, easy-read and interactive debrief tool was developed. The tool aims to support clients to discuss the incident as much or as little as they want, in a communication style which best suits them. The timing of when to go through the tool is person-centred, some clients wanting to debrief immediately after the incident and others needing more time to reflect upon the incident (one has been completed two weeks after an incident). The tool was developed with the input from a multidisciplinary team (MDT – made up of nursing, occupational therapy, speech and language therapy, psychology and psychiatry) to include multiple perspectives and create clear and accessible wording of questions.

'My Restraint Story' supports staff to facilitate a conversation with a client following the use of restrictive interventions. The story is usually completed with the client involved in restraint and a member of the support staff and is made up of three A3 laminated pages. The first page, 'What happened?', is a factual discussion of factors leading up to the restraint. Using symbols it supports the person to talk about five questions: where the person was; what they were doing; how they were feeling; how their body was feeling; where the person was in pain. Figure 24.1 shows how 'What happened?' appears in the toolkit.

The second page, 'Thinking about what happened', talks about what happened during the restraint. It asks: why the restraint happened; what staff did well/badly; if restraint helped the client. There is space for the client to share any thoughts they have about what could be done differently next time (by staff or client) to avoid future use of restraint. Asking the client

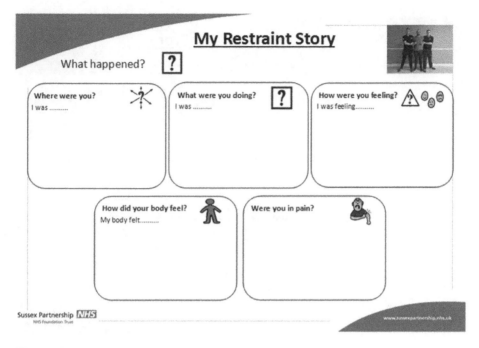

Figure 24.1 My Restraint Story, What happened?

their views on what staff did (whether good or bad) helps enable the conversation to not be driven by pre-determined goals of staff and allows the client/staff to reflect on the connections within their relationships that may have contributed to the use of restraint. It builds on the idea of circularity and that we are constantly influencing each other's behaviours. There is a strong focus to eliminate blame for the behaviour, supporting a discussion for looking into the context of the situation and to identify what the behaviour was trying to communicate. Figure 24.2 shows the format of the second page of the tool.

The third and last page, 'What about now?', revisits some of the questions asked on the first page and encourages the client to identify what support they need now to feel safe and secure. This checking-in page enables the client to express whether they feel composed, and if not, what they need to regain their composure. Figure 24.3 shows the format of this page.

When the tool has been completed, a picture of the finished tool can be taken and stored for recording purposes. A user guide has also been written to help all staff members to feel confident in using the tool. This includes some guidance around gaining a sense of the incident prior to using the tool and reading the client's communication support plan to make the tool as accessible as possible to the client. The stories are then stored in the central office at the ATU, so that they can be easily accessible to all support staff. The

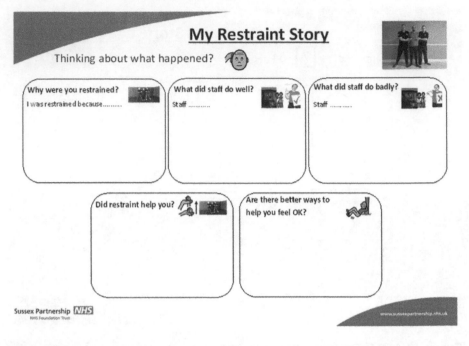

Figure 24.2   My Restraint Story, Thinking about what happened

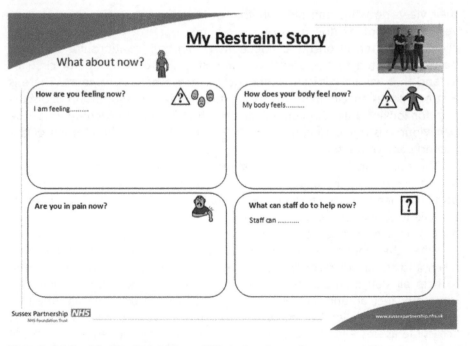

Figure 24.3   My Restraint Story, What about now?

story can also provide a reference to the client's perspective of the incident and can be shared (with the client's consent) at weekly MDT meetings. This allows the incidents to be discussed with the wider network of the client outside of the ATU (including family, friends, social care, community teams, etc.) so that multiple perspectives can offer insight to the situation and it offers further collaborative working for clients, currently or to help future thinking when they are discharged from the ATU.

Following observing clients at the ATU and listening to their comments after they had seen others being restrained, themes of confusion, fear and distress emerged. People who see or hear restraint may have painful memories and feelings of fearfulness (Mohr et al., 1998). Therefore, a sister tool was developed, the 'Seeing Restraint Story', for people who had witnessed someone being restrained. The tool follows the same format as the 'My Restraint Story'; however, questions have been adapted to ask about witnessing restraint at the ATU. This story can be used with more than one client (if they witness the same incident) and can facilitate the sharing of ideas/feelings/experiences from each other about the incident. Figure 24.4 shows the 'Seeing Restraint Story'.

To support each story, an image bank has been developed from a program called Boardmaker (Tobii Dynavox, 2018) and displayed in an A4-sized booklet.

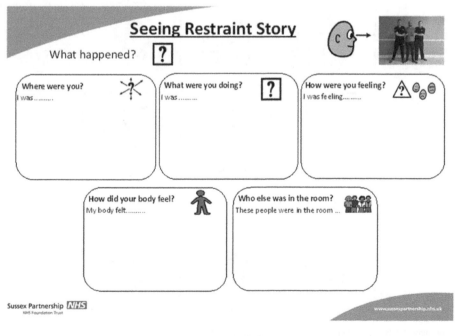

Figure 24.4   The Seeing Restraint Story page

Around 18–30 images support each question asked, which enables immediate access to picture symbols. These images can be unstuck from the image bank and placed onto the story. They follow 'Positive and Proactive Care' guidance (Department of Health, 2014), offering pictorial support for reporting if restraint was pain free, for the shortest time possible and the least restrictive. If the client does not wish to use images there is space to write their answer down. Offering a choice of communication styles enables the tool to be tailored to choice preference but can also reduce the demands of discussing these difficult experiences while still being able to hear the voice of the person who has been restrained. Figure 24.5 shows a page from the image bank.

Over recent years, there has been a drive to collaboratively work with people who use health services so that they can be involved in their own health,

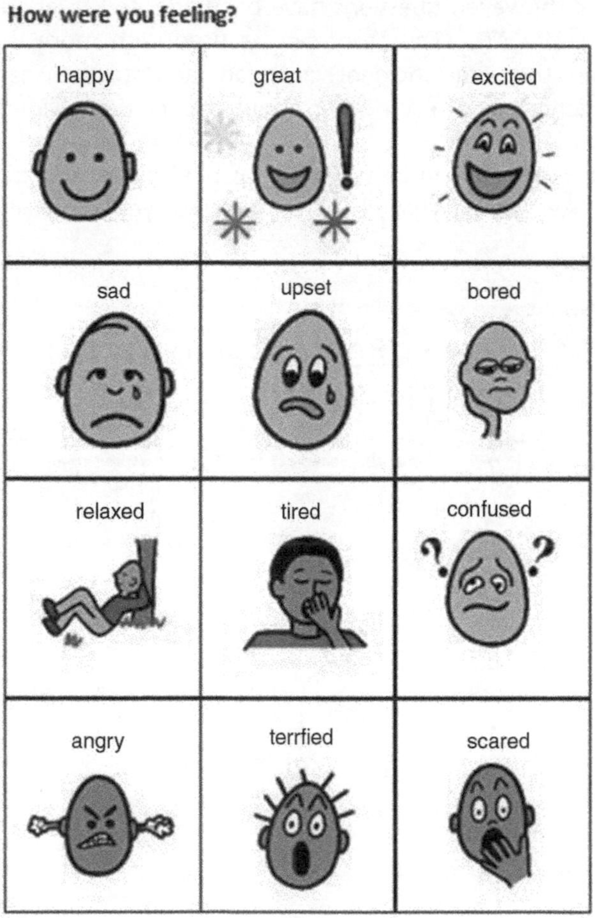

How were you feeling?

Figure 24.5 A page from the image bank[1]

care and treatment. NHS England's guidance 'Involving people in their own health and care' (2017), highlights the importance of this:

➤ It improves health and wellbeing (people make decisions and choices that optimise their physical and mental health).

➤ It improves quality of care (teams learn from feedback and people report greater satisfaction in the service).

➤ It improves financial sustainability and enables the efficient allocation of resources.

➤ It is a legal duty.

Service user involvement and collaborative working make people feel in control of their care and treatment and allows people to adapt their care and treatment to what matters to them (NHS England, 2017). This is even more important for people with learning disability, who have been described as being a group of people who are the 'most excluded, least independent and most likely to lack control in everyday life' (Department of Health, 2001). Feedback on the tools was gained from 'Powerful Trainers', award-winning experts with learning disabilities and unique insights, who raise awareness and help services to better understand the issues surrounding learning disability (Aldingbourne Trust, 2017). They reflected that incidents can indeed be hard to discuss and having them laid out in front of someone might make them easier to talk about. They liked the images to aid understanding and the choice of different styles of communication (images and writing). Further to this, a client at the ATU was particularly motivated to share their experience of using the tools. They have given consent for the following quotes to appear:

> I think they are very good and I am very proud of them [the completed tools]. Sometimes, I don't know why I have been restrained or why other people have been. They help me know that staff are ok when someone has tried to hurt them. I like the images, the images could help people who can't talk to understand what happened. It can be good to show other people what I thought about the restraint so they can understand my views and know what to do to calm me down.

The client also had some input around how the tools can be used in the best way:

> They [the tools] should be used straight after a restraint, only when they have calmed down, are talking quietly and not swearing. I would like to talk to a manager about

the restraint, because they are in charge of looking after everyone, but someone who knows me well is OK. It should be used in every hospital across the country.

The tools seem to have been useful in supporting people to discuss upsetting and difficult incidents in a way that is understandable to them. However, they also raise useful systemic and relational questions. For example, in what ways do the existence and use of these tools influence how the hospital staff understand the potential impact of being restrained or seeing others being restrained?

Box 24.1 Reflective questions on systemic approaches to debrief

- How do you think client views in debriefs might influence how the person is viewed within the service system?
- How might including more voices in a restraint story create a context which allows the 'facts' of a situation to be decided together, rather than just by professionals?
- What else could be done to include more voices and thicken the stories?

References

Aldingbourne Trust (2017). *Powerful Trainers*. Aldingbourne Trust. https://www.aldingbournetrust.org/projects.html (accessed 15 October 2017).

Bonner, G., Lowe, T., Rawcliffe, D. & Wellman, N. (2002). Trauma for all: A pilot study of the subjective experience of physical restraint for mental health inpatients and staff in the UK. *Journal of Psychiatric and Mental Health Nursing*, 9(4), 465–473.

Department of Health (2001). *Valuing People: A New Strategy for Learning Disability for the 21st Century*. London: Department of Health.

Department of Health (2012). *Transforming Care: A national response to Winterbourne View Hospital*. https://assets.publishing.service.gov.uk/government/uploads/system/uploads/attachment_data/file/213215/final-report.pdf (accessed 1 February 2018).

Department of Health (2014). *Positive and Proactive Care: Reducing the Need for Restrictive Interventions*. London: Department of Health.

Department of Health. (2015). *Mental Health Act, 1983; Code of Practice*. Norwich: The Stationery Office.

Mohr, W.K., Mahon, M.M. & Noone, M.J. (1998). A restraint on restraints: The need to reconsider restrictive interventions. *Arch Psychiatry Nursing*, 12, 95–106.

National Institute for Health and Care Excellence (NICE) (2015). *Violence and Aggression: Short Term Management in Mental Health, Health and Community Settings. NICE Guidelines [NG10].* London: Department of Health.

NHS England (2017). Involving people in their own health and care: Statutory guidance for clinical commissioning groups and NHS England. UK: NHS England.

Sequeira, H. & Halstead, S. (2002). Control and restraint in the UK: Service user perspectives. *The Journal of Forensic Practice,* 4(1), 9–18.

Sutton, D., Webster, S. & Wilson, M. (2014). *Debriefing following Seclusion and Restraint. A Summary of Relevant Literature.* Auckland: Te Pou Te Whakaaro Nui: the National Centre of Mental Health Research, Information and Workforce Development.

Notes

1   The Picture Communication Symbols ©1981–2018 by Tobii Dynavox. All Rights Reserved Worldwide. Used with permission.
Boardmaker® is a trademark of Tobii Dynavox.

25

Prejudices

Victoria Jones

Accessible summary

- When two or more people are together they have an effect on each other.

- All our ideas, beliefs, theories, stories, feelings and experiences can be thought of as prejudices.

- Prejudices can be positive and negative.

- Prejudices are things to find out about and make useful, not something to ignore or hide from.

- If we know what our prejudices are then we can try and do something about them.

The movement into second-order cybernetics emphasised that we cannot work with people without becoming a part of the system. Campbell described this as an 'emphasis upon the therapist as an active, necessarily biased, co-constructor of therapeutic realities' (Campbell, 2003, p. 18). This recognises that through the process of observation we influence and alter what it is we are looking at.

Imagine I walk into a room where someone is distressed and their behaviour is becoming a challenge to others. I can anticipate that my presence will have some effect upon the dynamics in the room. My potential effect could depend upon my background, training, experience, relationship with each person in the room, expectations, feelings that day, or even general health. It is quite possible that a different person walking into the same situation might make a very different impact. Thus, rather than try to work in a way that attempts to ignore or minimise the effect that we make on people and their systems, what we really should try to do is identify, name and embrace the ways in which we may be influencing a system or situation. This enables us to make further efforts to explore and predict those factors to make them useful to the human system that we are seeking to help. It also helps us to name and better manage those things which are not helping.

This challenge in second-order approaches was articulated by Cecchin et al. (1994) when they referred to the biases that impact on the way we interact with a system as 'prejudices'. This is a way of considering the thoughts and ideas that we each bring to a situation, whether consciously or not. They described prejudice as 'the sets of fantasies, ideas, accepted historical facts, models, theories, personal feelings, moods, unrecognised loyalties – in fact, any pre-existing thought that contributes to one's views, perceptions and actions' (p. 8).

Prejudices incorporate any fixed view, idea or knowledge that a person holds. Thus the term applies to both the positive and negative things that influence us.

This challenges the more common view of prejudice as detrimentally discriminatory and invites us to seek out our as-yet-unacknowledged prejudices. This perspective frees us up to consider all the aspects of our thinking without being caught in a cycle of confusion, guilt or doubt. It enables us to embrace the ideas we hold in a new way. As a result, the exploration of our own prejudices can become more of a dip into a treasure trove than a woeful trawl through our very own Pandora's box. That is not to say that we should hold our prejudices without undue care and attention. Part of our task as citizens is to ensure that we identify when our views and ideas challenge or negatively affect our capacity to be useful to others. Our ethical and professional responsibility in such a situation would be to seek support to manage the potential for detrimental effects on the people we are engaged with, our colleagues and ourselves. This could entail seeking mentorship, raising the matter in supervision or undertaking further training, as well as ensuring our practice is regularly reflective, reflexive and recursive.

Personal prejudices

Our own personal biases might stem from ideas or beliefs in our family of origin and our lived experiences. They are likely to be linked to the cultural norms that we experienced growing up, the social characteristics that we identify with and our own experiences of belonging, oppression, privilege and intersectionality (also see 'Diversity IS GRACE', Chapter 20). It is important to notice that our prejudices and the prominence that we afford them may vary across time, context and who we are in a relationship with at any given time.

Box 25.1 Reflective questions on my own prejudices

- What sense do I make of my own gender, race, religion, impairments, abilities, culture, class, ethnicity, education and sexuality?

- What other prejudices (views, ideas and knowledge) might I hold?

- Are there prejudices that others would claim I hold?

- Which prejudices stem from my family of origin (childhood family); family of creation (the family I share my adult life with); interests and hobbies; beliefs and values?

- Which of my prejudices do I value more than others? Why? (What are my prejudices about my prejudices?)

- What might they each mean for the work that I do?

- In what way might I be able to make them useful to the systems (individuals, teams and organisations) that I work with?

- What views, ideas and knowledge do I hold about 'learning disability' and people who have been labelled with it?

- How can I make best use of support and supervision to help me explore and effectively work with all of my prejudices?

The Daisy Model

Developed as part of Coordinated Management of Meaning, this tool uses the shape of a daisy to help us consider all the factors that may be influencing a conversation or event (CMM, Pearce Associates, 2004). It can be used to help us look at what we bring to the front of our thinking in conversations with ourselves and others. Each petal of the daisy represents a bias or prejudice that may be influencing the way that we act. Complete the daisy in Figure 25.1 to consider the wealth of personal prejudices, ideas and biases that you will take to your next day at work.

In each petal write a prejudice, bias, idea, story, or other factor that influences who you are and how you are:

Figure 25.1   Using the CMM Daisy Model to consider the personal prejudices I take to work

Professional prejudices

Prejudices also arise from our professional training. When we have worked hard to become a particular type of professional and to qualify as a member of that group it is easy not to notice the prejudices that we have absorbed and accepted along the way. If we do not take time to consider what it is that influences us it can be quite a surprise when they come to the fore. For example, as a newly qualified learning disability nurse I was employed in a residential service run by adult social services. I believed that my prejudices were all about empowerment and quality of life and were entirely compatible with the team. However, I was surprised that my attention and subsequent advocacy for change rapidly centred on the menu that included no fruit or vegetables when 90 per cent of the people living there regularly took medication for constipation. It was news to me that I had taken on board my training about good health and wellbeing to such an extent that this was something I felt needed prioritising. The challenge for me was to notice that whilst it may well have been a beneficial intervention, what brought it to light was my prejudices, and I had a responsibility to explore how best to make that useful in collaboration with the people I was supporting.

This example of a professional prejudice also highlights the challenge of multi-professional team working. I wonder what a new 'resident', speech therapist, social worker or psychologist might have settled on as their focus of concern. Individually reflecting on our own conscious, and unconscious, hard-earned professional prejudices is crucial if we are to be able to make them optimally useful. It can also avoid the risk of imposing them on others. Taking time to articulate the things that influence us by writing a 'position statement' that incorporates our own current thinking, views, theoretical influences, ways of working and future directions is one way of doing this. Alternatively, you might add 'professional petals' to the daisy you completed in Figure 25.1. These can form part of an ongoing professional portfolio and can also be useful when putting together applications for posts.

Of course, if everyone in a team brought in their own completed daisy models there would be multiple overlaps and connections made between them. You could imagine that this might create a chrysanthemum of many petals with the dynamics of the team happening at the centre of the flower. When working in teams it is critical that we creatively explore how we might manage a 'conversation' between our prejudices to promote the wishes and best interests of the people we serve. Developing and sustaining relationships and a culture that can facilitate such dialogue is arguably the crux of effective multidisciplinary and inter-agency working. One possible technique for this would be to hold a reflecting conversation. For example, two members of the team discuss an issue or concern in front of the rest of the team before then taking a turn to listen to the other members of the team reflect on their thoughts and ideas about what they heard in the initial discussion. Finally, the whole team have a full group discussion to see where the conversation and thinking has gone (also refer to 'Reflecting Conversations', Chapter 26).

Person-centred approaches are central to our current health and social care policies (Health Foundation, 2014). A necessary attribute of this is the ability to be authentically ourselves in our interactions with others (McCance et al., 2013). Consequently, it is important that we strive to know ourselves and the things that influence us. The concept of prejudices offered by Cecchin et al. (1994) invites us to embrace all the things that contribute to that sense of self and to seek out whatever may influence our capacity to optimally engage with each person we meet.

References

Campbell, D. (2003). The mutiny and the bounty: The place of Milan ideas today. *Australia and New Zealand Journal of Family Therapy*, 24(1), 15–25.

Cecchin, G., Lane, G. & Ray, W. (1994). *The Cybernetics of Prejudices in the Practice of Psychotherapy*. London: Karnac.

Health Foundation (2014). *Person-Centred Care Made Simple*. London: Health Foundation.

McCance, T., Gribben, B., McCormack, B. & Laird, E. (2013). Promoting person-centred practice within acute care: The impact of culture and context on a facilitated practice development programme. *International Practice Development Journal*, 3(1), 2, 1–17.

Pearce Associates. (2004). *Using CMM 'The Coordinated Management of Meaning'*. www.pearceassociates.com/essays/cmm_seminar.pdf (accessed 25 February 2018).

26

Reflecting Conversations – Separating Talk and Listening: Using Reflecting Conversation to Create New Understandings with People Affected by Learning Disability and their Families and Networks

Sarah Coles and Selma Rikberg Smyly

Accessible summary

- Separating talking and listening by using a reflecting team approach can create new understandings of the problem.

- Finding ways to talk together so that everyone can be listened to is important.

- We include examples of how reflecting conversation is used in different ways and how it can create shifts in meanings.

Our context

We are clinical psychologists who worked together within the context of an NHS multidisciplinary team for adults affected by learning disability. In our work with this client group we found that referrals were often made for so-called 'challenging behaviour' which covered any amount and variety of distress experienced by either the person involved and/or their carers. Given Gergen's view that 'there are no truths, only more or less helpful ways of seeing the problem' (1994, p.33) our preferred way of working was to use different kinds of reflecting conversations with individuals, families and staff teams. This enabled sharing of how the referred 'challenging behaviour' was experienced by the people involved and the different meanings created around this behaviour. Our preferred way of working was to use different kinds of reflecting conversations with individuals, families and staff teams to share an understanding of how this 'challenging behaviour' was experienced by the people involved and the different meanings created around this behaviour. From this type of shared conversation new ideas emerged about why someone might be distressed and what different ways of helping might look like.

What do we do when we reflect?

We fluctuate between interviewing our clients in the room and then pausing the interview to talk with each other in front of them (separating the talking and listening) to generate different meanings around the behaviour of concern. The method of using reflective teams in sessions is an important part of social constructionist practice where a non-expert position, multiple perspectives and the co-creation of alternative stories can be modelled (Andersen, 1987, 1991). The separating of talking and listening offers the opportunity for inner conversation to be heard and shared together with the outer conversation (Andersen, 1987, 1991). A detailed example of how we have used this is given in Rikberg Smyly and Coles, 2017.

Our intention is to try to create enough 'news of difference' (Bateson, 1972) with the aim of enabling shifts in thinking, and different ways of seeing and understanding. Being mindful to use valuing and respectful language, we might talk to each other about what we have noticed, or how the context is impacting on our understanding. We try to situate what we say in the language that has been used in the room. We might ask each other questions such as: where do you think that idea came from? What was it you heard in the conversation that made you wonder that? Following the reflections the clients (this could be a combination of the referred client, family members and/or staff team members) are invited to comment on what they have heard and how this may have resonated with them. This process can be repeated a number of times within the meeting. It is a way of hearing each other's point of view and understandings in a tentative and transparent way. The clients are always free to accept or disregard the reflections if they don't fit or make sense to them.

What does reflecting conversation look like?

We decide between us how we will use each other in the session. One of us will be the interviewer and the other is the reflecting person (RP). The interviewer talks directly with the invited clients; the RP usually sits slightly outside the conversation and listens to the interview without contributing to the conversation between invited clients. If we are lucky to have more than the two of us present we use a reflecting team, in which case the interviewer would sit outside of the reflecting conversation.

If possible we try to ensure that we have more clients (or at least equal numbers) in the room than clinicians. About halfway through the meeting (which usually lasts and hour and a half), the interviewer turns to the RP and has a conversation the clients listen to. The interviewer then turns back to clients and they have a chance to comment. We might ask the clients to comment on what surprised them, or resonated for them. The RP does not usually speak directly to the clients.

Preparing for sessions

We usually have a conversation with the referrer on the phone (as we perceive the referrer to be our client – they are the ones inviting us into their system). In this conversation we think about what is going to be most useful in terms of starting work together. This initial talk also enables us to think about who the relevant people might be to invite to a first session (in terms of understanding the dilemmas raised in the referral). This might be the referrer, the individual, the family, and the staff team from the residential and/or day service. We usually ask about different ideas across the system of concern and what the client's view might be about the problem. We also discuss the organisation of the first meeting in terms of practicalities such as venue and time. If we are including the person with the learning disability we will often meet with them (before holding a larger meeting) to think with them about the meeting and how best to support them in terms of who they think needs to be there, what their view is and how we can ensure their voice is heard.

Following these steps, before we go into a session the interviewer and RP use the pre-session template (Rikberg Smyly, 2012) to enable us to think about the referral and the questions we want to ask in session. In particular we focus on differences in context, as well as meanings and beliefs around the referral and the possibly different understandings of the problem and expectations of help (Reder & Fredman, 1996). The first session usually focuses on what different people in the network think about the problem and what ideas they have about what help might look like.

Conversations with the networks about relationships to help

Our intention during the interview is to begin to ask questions relating to the ideas we have generated about the referral, the aim being that these questions give us a sense of the different beliefs and understandings within the system of concern. However, it is usually helpful to start with the position of hearing and witnessing the current difficulties our clients are facing before asking any specific questions about the relationship to help.

Throughout the session we are aware that together the questions we ask and the reflecting conversation begin to open up different ways of understanding the problem. Some of the most helpful questions we consider and reflect on cover the relationship to help (Reder & Fredman, 1996), such as:

➤ Who is most/least concerned about the problem?

➤ What has led to the referral being made now?

➤ What kind of change and/or help is the client/team hoping for?

➤ Have they had input from psychology before? What was it like?

➤ What is the client's view about the problem?

➤ What is happening at times when the problem is around?

➤ What changes have there been for the staff team and the client?

Shifting meanings and beliefs through context

Carter and McGoldrick (1989) noted how people can often experience problems at times of significant change in their life cycle stages. We've noticed this in our client group, and we've also noticed that the context of this is often lost. Stories are told, behaviour is interpreted and explained by others rather than through hearing the voice of the person with learning disability about their own life. This can result in rather thin descriptions (Morgan, 2000; Scior & Lynggaard, 2006) of the client's lived experiences, for example that it is the learning disability that is causing the issue rather than that distress is being created by life cycle transitions.

During both the interview and reflecting part of our meetings with clients we are thinking about how changing the context can lead to different ideas and meanings being given. We ask questions about how ideas have come about and what has influenced them (i.e. family beliefs or the cultural context).

For example, a man in his 50s was referred for 'challenging behaviour' by his home manager. We were particularly interested in the use of language in the referral and wondered what the meaning of this behaviour was for the gentleman and his network. Later as the conversation developed we found out that his day service (which he had attended for 30 years) had been changed without his consultation. This was not seen as relevant by the staff team, but had deeply affected the man as he felt this was his job, and he was missing seeing a number of important friends. The distress or anger was being conceptualised as part of the learning disability, or free floating, rather than associated with losing something important. In the session, rather than 'telling the team this' I (SC) reflected with the interviewer that I remembered when my dad had lost his job and the effect that this had on him in relation to his mood. This was made as a tentative offering which was picked up on by staff. A conversation followed about how this could be similar for the person they were supporting. Recognising the context meant that the staff team could think of ways to support the client including working on a life story book with him, and finding out different ways for him to keep in touch with the people he missed from the centre.

In another systemic consultation concerning a referral of a client in a group home who was seen to be unable to deal with a recent bereavement, the staff team were encouraged to explore their ideas and beliefs about how one grieved; different cultural norms; and the acceptable ways of expressing grief. It transpired that some staff members found conversations about bereavement particularly distressing and felt the client brought up the subject of death to upset them. Some held a view that to 'be strong was not to talk about it' whereas others felt that it was too close to their own experiences and they wanted to protect themselves from remembering their own experiences of grief. In our reflections we wondered about the person with learning disabilities' view of talking or not talking, and what death meant to them. How did it fit with their family's view of death? How did it fit with the client's level of ability and their conceptual or developmental understanding of death, or their spiritual or religious views? Opening out the conversation made the different explanations about the client's response to death more explicit and more understandable. It also highlighted the different and varied expectations and responses the staff held. As a result of our conversations the staff team felt the client would benefit from being supported by a couple of staff who felt comfortable talking to him about his grief (Rikberg Smyly, 2009).

Working with just one therapist in the room

Sometimes we work on our own, for example, with a person with a learning disability and their chosen support worker. At these times we might still separate the talking and listening, for example by interviewing the client and inviting the support worker to reflect with us on this conversation. Our intention might be to help expand the meanings of the words used by the client. Finding out how others might interpret such conversations adds more possible perspectives to the conversation. Many of our clients may only use one or two different words which may typically hold a whole host of different meanings (Cardone & Hilton, 2006). This is where local knowledge may be very helpful to increase our understanding of the possible meanings implied in such conversations

Final reflections

We have found that by working in a way that promotes multiple understandings of experiences and where the voices of clients, networks and professionals are more equally heard and shared, it becomes possible to facilitate conversations that enable changes in understanding and action to take place.

Box 26.1 A reflecting conversation exercise

You will need at least three people for this task. Think about someone you are currently working with. One person acts as an interviewer and asks the second some questions about the referral as outlined in the interview section above (Rikberg Smyly, 2012). After 10 to 15 minutes the interviewer turns to the RP (reflecting person) and the two of you have a conversation on your thoughts about what they have heard. The RP can ask themselves the following questions: what ideas did I have about what was being said? What other questions did I have? The interviewer shifts back to supervisee: what resonated for them? How have their ideas changed/how do they feel now? Who do they want to meet with and why?

References

Andersen, T. (1987). The reflecting team: Dialogue and meta-dialogue in clinical work. *Family Process*, 26, 415–428.

Andersen, T. (ed.) (1991). *The Reflecting Team: Dialogues and Dialogues about Dialogues*. New York: Norton.

Bateson, G. (1972). *Steps to an Ecology of Mind*. New York: Ballantine Books.

Cardone, D. & Hilton, A. (2006). Engaging people with learning disabilities in systemic therapy. In S. Baum & H. Lynggaard (eds), *Intellectual Disabilities: A Systemic Approach* (pp. 83–98). London: Karnac.

Carter, B. & McGoldrick, M. (1989). *The Changing Family Life-Cycle: A Framework to Family Therapy*. 2nd edition. Boston, MA: Ally & Bacon.

Gergen, K.J. (1994). *Realities and Relationships: Soundings in Social Construction*. Cambridge, MA: Harvard University Press.

Morgan, A. (2000). *What is Narrative Therapy?* Adelaide: Dulwich Centre Publication.

Reder, P. & Fredman, G. (1996). The relationship to help: Interacting beliefs about the treatment process. *Clinical Psychology and Psychiatry*, 1(3), 457–467.

Rikberg Smyly, S. (2009). Working systemically with people with learning disabilities. In H. Beinart et al. (eds), *Clinical Psychology in Practice* (pp. 164–174). Chichester: John Wiley & Sons.

Rikberg Smyly, S. (2012). How do we know what to ask? Using pre session hypothesising to develop systemic questions. *Clinical Psychology and People with Learning Disabilities*, 10(2), 4–11.

Rikberg Smyly, S. & Coles, S. (2017). Working with two consultants. Reflecting conversations to create new ways to go on in staff teams. In G. Fredman, A. Papadopoulou & E. Worwood (eds), *Collaborative Consultation in Mental Health: Guidelines for the New Consultant* (pp. 135–151). Oxon and New York: Routledge.

Scior, K. & Lynggaard, H. (2006). New stories of intellectual disabilities: A narrative approach. In S. Baum & H. Lynggaard (eds), *Intellectual Disabilities: A Systemic Approach* (pp. 100–119). London: Karnac.

27

Reframing

Victoria Jones

Accessible summary

- Reframing is about offering people different ways to make sense of something.

- Reframing can help people, services and families find hope and believe that things can change.

- Reframing is not about persuading people that staff/professionals know better.

- Reframing should not stop us from thinking about how to keep people safe and well.

Reframing involves taking a concept and looking at it from a different angle or perspective in such a way that the meaning of the original actually shifts and is understood in a new way (Watzlawick et al., 1974). Metaphorically, if the frame around a piece of art is replaced it can highlight new colours, tints and aspects, enabling the viewer to see it with new eyes even though the painting itself has not been altered.

Reframing, then, involves changing the way a situation or behaviour is considered or viewed, either emotionally, conceptually or contextually, so that the meaning of the behaviour also changes. It is not just about trying to create a new truth but supporting clients, families and ourselves to see the same thing in a different way so that we find a new understanding of it. In this way the behaviour becomes something that people can begin to accept or cope with more readily. Reframing can also help us to find ways to make behaviours useful.

   A key consideration for successful reframing is that it is the way the situation or behaviour is understood that shifts rather than the behaviour itself. In this way reframing is a good example of second-order change, where it is the meaning and the way we make sense of it that has changed even though the situation is much the same. That said, once someone has made a shift in their understanding it may make it possible for the behaviours themselves to more readily change even though that was not the goal of the reframe.

   To make sense of this take a look again at the classic picture we previously encountered in Chapter 22. In Figure 27.1 do you see a young woman looking away or an old woman with a big nose? What is it that helps you to see both?

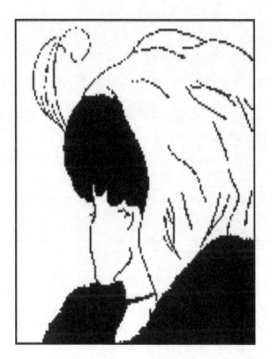

Figure 27.1   A classic optical illusion that demonstrates the power of perspective and the potential for reframing

(Hill, 1915)

How can we make reframing useful in services for people with learning disabilities?

Reframing can help us to show people their strengths and resilience: consider Jake, a new father with a nine-month-old daughter, who speaks with you about his fears that he might neglect his child in the same way that he was neglected before he was taken into care as a young child. He is worried that he has never been shown how to be a good dad and he finds it hard to learn new things because of his learning disability. Whilst you could agree with him and raise concerns that his daughter may be at risk, you may also seize this opportunity to reframe his worry as him showing a huge capacity to be a protective, concerned and loving father who is already problem solving about how to be good enough for his child. This shifts his own concerns about perceived weakness into strengths and opportunities. Reframing enables you to identify not simply that he wishes to look after his daughter well, but also that he has shown that he can share his worries in a way that enables both he and his daughter to receive appropriate support.

Reframing can also help us to see behaviours as more logical and 'sense-able'. By changing the context of a behaviour, or its frame, we can find ways to make our quirks less misunderstood, or possibly even valuable. John Lee Cronin had a penchant for what he called his 'crazy socks' and was always looking for shops supplying new pairs to add to his collection. For John, socks helped him to communicate his personality and his mood. Working with his dad they reframed this interest and co-founded a business, John's Crazy Socks, with a mission to 'spread happiness through socks'. At the time of writing their online catalogue offers over 1200 pairs of socks and their ethically oriented company employs other disabled people (www.johnscrazysocks. com).

Another reframe that could be easily overlooked involves shining a light on supporting the recognition of diversity and our understanding of the specific effects of a person's impairment. I once supported a woman, Claire, who had a severe learning difficulty in addition to a rare neurological condition called Moebius syndrome. Claire was declined a place in an under-resourced course that was staffed largely by volunteers because she 'doesn't smile much' and 'appears aggressive and confrontational'. It took very little time to educate the service manager that due to her impairment effects she was physically unable to make facial expressions. Denying her a service on this basis was discriminatory. As a result, Claire was offered a place on the course, although it left us to debate the matter of whether she would want to access a service that expected its recipients to be happy and smile a lot.

Some fundamental questions in our reframing repertoire should also include: 'If this person did not "have" a learning disability what difference would it make to our response and what we consider possible?' closely followed by 'What difference *should* it then make, to them and me, that they are considered to "have" a learning disability?' It is important not to overlook health and safety considerations that may impact upon a person and the people around them but responses should be the least restrictive option (The Department for Constitutional Affairs, 2007).

Reframing links with the concept of person-centred practice which seeks to explore ways to celebrate individuality, rights, strengths, choice, autonomy and community networks and to provide creative solutions for support (Cambridge & Carnaby, 2005; Sanderson & Lewis, 2012). These emphases make it an ideal approach when seeking to deliver both co-production and personalisation. Specifically, the 'reputations' exercise outlined below invites us to find positive ways to reframe an individual's 'negative reputations' and to consider whether there is some context, or frame, in which their behaviour might be seen as positive. This is because such reputations may be out of date, inaccurate and dehumanising, and restrict access to opportunities and choices.

When searching for ways to reframe a negative reputation into a positive one it may help to imagine that you are talking about the annoying habits or negative traits of a good friend or describing someone who might just be listening over your shoulder. It is important to strive to be positive, to avoid trying to apportion blame and use appropriate, valuing language to describe the person. In this way reputations, whether of colleagues or clients, can be re-visioned. For example, 'She's really nosey' can become 'She has her finger on the pulse and if you need to know something talk to her'; 'He's lazy' might suit 'He has a brilliant capacity for relaxation and not getting flustered'; and 'She never sleeps' might be 'She would be great working night shifts'.

Box 27.1 Reputations exercise

The reputations tool helps people to think about the negative things that someone may say or do, talk about it when these things happen, and then for each negative ask three questions:

1. Are there situations where the negative can be seen as a positive thing? If yes, this is something to record and celebrate as something that is appreciated about the person.

2. Does the negative reflect something that is important to the person? If yes, record it as something that is important to that person.

3. Consider if the negative sometimes really is a negative. If it is, what should other people know or do to support the person when this is happening? Record this as a requirement for their good support.

This exercise was developed by Helen Sanderson Associates and The Learning Community for Person Centered Practices (TLCPCP, 2011); more information about it can be found at:

www.facs.nsw.gov.au/download?file=590649

For ideas and a wide range of other person-centred thinking and practice tools explore this site:

www.helensandersonassociates.co.uk

In both reframing and creating positive reputations it is important to check with people that there is currency for them in the new idea. This is not an exercise in finding a new truth or persuading them to accept professional ideas but rather in seeking a more useful way to make sense for now. Jointly recognising that their relationship to the problem has shifted can often serve to help people come together with a renewed willingness and energy to find longer term solutions.

Box 27.2 Reflective questions on reframing

Identify situations in your work where it might be useful to be able to think differently through reframing someone's actions or behaviour.

Are there ways in which that person's behaviour makes sense or can be seen as positive?

How might you share these ideas with your team?

References

Cambridge, P. & Carnaby, S. (2005). *Person Centred Planning and Care Management with People with Learning Disabilities*. London: Jessica Kingsley Publishers.

The Department for Constitutional Affairs. (2007). *The Mental Capacity Act 2005 Code of Practice*. London: Crown Copyright.

Helen Sanderson Associates – resources for person centred practice and training. www.helensandersonassociates.co.uk (accessed 28 February 2018).

Helen Sanderson Associates and The Learning Community for Person Centered Practices. (2011). *Reputations Exercise*. www.facs.nsw.gov.au/download?file=590649 (accessed 12 September 2018).

Hill, W. (1915). My wife and my mother-in-law. *Puck*, 16(11), Nov.

John Lee Cronin's Sock Shop (n.d.). www.johnscrazysocks.com (accessed 28 February 2018).

Sanderson, H. & Lewis, J. (2012). *A Practical Guide to Delivering Personalisation*. London: Jessica Kingsley Publishers.

Watzlawick, P., Weakland, J. & Fisch, R. (1974). *Change: Principles of Problem Formation and Problem Resolution*. New York: W.W. Norton.

28

Relational Reflexivity: Talking About How We Do Talking and Being Together

Victoria Jones

Accessible summary

- It is very useful to plan with people how we are going to talk together.

- You can do this before, during and after a meeting.

- This is especially important when supporting people who are not used to being listened to.

- When we get this right we are being respectful and person-centred.

Relational reflexivity is:

> the intention, desire, processes and practices through which therapists and clients explicitly engage one another in coordinating their resources so as to create a relationship with therapeutic potential. This would involve initiating, responding to, and developing opportunities to consider, explore, experiment with and elaborate the ways in which they relate.

> (Burnham, 2005, p. 4)

This is especially important when we are supporting individuals whose voice and power has been diminished or not attended to as is so often the case for women, men, girls and boys who have been labelled with a learning disability. By working together to build a guiding framework for where the conversation and activities are going you are much more likely to be truly collaborative and co-productive in your practice. Table 28.1 is a development of the work of Burnham (2005); Haydon-Laurelut (2016) and the myriad techniques of person-centred thinking and practice (e.g. the excellent Helen

Table 28.1   Relational reflexivity – collaborating about engagement

Theme	Goal	Example
Initial appointments	Inviting the other into a person-centred process of partnership and collaboration from the first contact.	Accessible letters and initial contact. Timing to suit the individual – not first thing if they aren't good in the morning, or close to their monthly depot injection or a stressful contact visit etc. Location to suit the individual in terms of, for example, access, travel, comfort, ambience. Considering who should be invited with the individual themselves.
First contact	Making a relationship with the person in front of you, not the person on the referral.	Holding referral information cautiously in your mind. Being curious about who this person is and what we can make together. 'As we haven't met before is there anything you think I should do to help us work together well?'
Warming the context	Making it less scary, increasing readiness of you both to engage, helping people feel ready and able to join in.	Smiling; greeting; getting ready; explaining what is coming; welcoming; running through what might happen; inviting rather than telling. 'How was your journey here today?'
Questions about questions	Involve the person in the direction of questions rather than imposing them. This achieves a better fit for them; is more person-centred; encourages engagement.	'Shall I ask you about "when" this will happen or "if" this will happen?' 'Shall we start with this or that?' 'Who wants to speak about this first?' 'What might make it harder for us to talk about when that happened?'
Relationship to help	For us all to explore how we like to receive/offer assistance and what we expect to offer and receive from this episode of care/support/intervention.	'Whose idea was it that we met today?' 'How hopeful are you that we can change this together?' 'Who has been most useful to you in the past? If they were to give me tips about helping you, what do you think they would say?' 'How would we know if this was working for you?'

Theme	Goal	Example
Preparing listeners to respond to what they hear	We all listen to diminished voices more effectively. To show the speaker that you are also on their side.	This is especially useful when asked to talk *to* someone about something while the person requesting is listening in. 'While Rob and I are talking, can you listen out for the things that you weren't expecting to hear?' 'Can you listen for the good things/for what she finds really hard to cope with?'
Preparing people to hear good things about themselves	To be able to positively connote and celebrate individual strengths and successes in a way that people can really hear and believe.	'Do you think we could fill this note page with what you are good at or do we need a flip chart? Which would you like better?' 'In a minute we are going to hear all about what you are great at...' 'What do you think she most likes about you? Shall I ask her now or later?'
Responding to emotions	Ensuring that our responses to each other's distress fits with what people need and find useful.	'When you have tears in your eyes would you like me to offer you a tissue or keep talking?' 'You talk about being scared. Shall we focus on the fear or would you like to explore when you have been brave?'
Negotiating approach, method and techniques	Not imposing ways of working; pursuing co-production of outputs.	'I think it might be helpful for us to do a family tree. Is that OK?' 'Do you have an idea about how we might do it?' 'Would you like to draw it or me?' 'How shall we record the men and the women?' 'I have an idea that there are things that make things harder when you have a learning disability? What do you think? Does that make sense for you and your life?'

Theme	Goal	Example
Pace	Recognising that we all experience time differently and have different capacities to engage over time.	'What would you like to start with today?' 'Tell me when you think it's nearly time to finish today.' 'Should we make our meeting longer or shorter next time?'
Keeping it going	Reducing stress and assisting engagement.	Using social stories to prepare for your meeting. Offering contact in between meetings, e.g. about future appointments, conversation planning. Be clear about the structure of each session and your likely work together. 'Next time shall we do things the same or differently?'
Inclusive communication	Accessible and inclusive communication that values every person's communication style, voice and contribution.	Encouraging everyone to use communication methods and language that can include every person in the room. Considering voice tone; speed; pitch; formality; and the duration of each episode of speech. These all play a part in meeting cognitive needs but also in aurally holding and containing the communication, the way that human sounds can make a space feel welcoming, supportive and safe. Agreeing a core vocabulary that is meaningful to everyone – 'When we get together should we call it a planning meeting or a chat? What's the difference?' Keeping meeting records in an accessible format. 'Shall we use words or pictures for our record?'
Being cautious about choices	Not overloading or over-tiring someone with our enthusiasm for collaboration.	'Do you find it tiring when I keep asking you to make choices?' 'How many decisions can you make in one hour?' 'If I give you three things to choose from is that a bit too much?'

Sanderson Associates website) and explores how we can collaborate with others to engage more effectively.

The relationally reflexive themes identified in Table 28.1 can help us to continuously develop a wider range of techniques that enable us to appropriately scaffold the interactions that we invite each person to join us in.

I believe that the most effective and truly person-centred practitioners are those who never give up an opportunity to seek a way to collaborate with people in the process of exploring how they would like to be engaged. This offers us all many opportunities to explore creativity in our practice. More fundamentally, however, it is both a respectful and a relationally ethical stance for us to take whenever we share moments with people whose voice is so often undermined and diminished.

References

Burnham, J. (2005). Relational reflexivity: A tool for socially constructing therapeutic relationships. In C. Flaskas, B. Mason & A. Perlesz (eds) *The Space Between: Experience, Context, and Process in the Therapeutic Relationship* (pp. 1–17). London: Karnac Books.

Haydon-Laurelut, M. (2016). Systemic therapy and autistic spectrum conditions. *Context*, 144, April, 18–20.

Helen Sanderson Associates. www.helensandersonassociates.co.uk (accessed 5 April 2018).

To Conclude

Accessible summary

- We're all in this together.
- Keep asking questions.
- Dare to dream.

In one way or another we all experience this idea we call 'learning disability' and together construct the meaning that we individually and collectively afford it. Our experiences are wide and varied: maybe as people who have been labelled with 'it'; pregnant women invited to screen for 'it'; families with beloved members who live with 'it'; as playmates; employees; taxpayers; and citizens. The list is endless. From a systemic perspective moment by moment, interaction by interaction, word by word and story by story we are all collectively creating and recreating this concept we think of as 'learning disability'. Considering it this way, we are all people *with* learning disability, each of us is a person *with* 'it' and this book is about you and me.

Lannamann suggested that the path to change and the avoidance of maintaining power imbalances is not through actually finding the answers to the questions that most challenge us but in being loud and clear about shaping, refining and articulating the questions that explore our own ideologies and constrain what it is possible for us to be curious about.

> When we see the constraints that limit our choices we are aware of power relations; when we see only choices we live in and reproduce power.
>
> (Lannamann, 1991, p. 198).

When thinking about CMM theory, Holmgren described *game mastery* as a willingness to engage others in making new discourses and finding 'another story based on other rules and moral assumptions than the ones they have followed until now' (Holmgren, 2004, p. 99). We think the systemic ideas in this book offer an insight into how we can develop our skills and abilities to work with others in this way. We warmly invite you to practise game mastery and be part of creating a context and culture where the 'rules' about learning disability can bend, evolve and be challenged; where the moral order and 'how it is' can be questioned; where we can voice our curiosity about what is unsaid or unheard; and where we can play devil's advocate and take delight in the fireworks and sparks of new understanding and changes that are generated – for ourselves, our organisations and our communities – as a result.

References

Holmgren, A. (2004). Saying, doing and making: Teaching CMM theory. *Human Systems: The Journal of Systemic Consultation and Management*, 15(2), 89–100.
Lannamann, J. (1991). Interpersonal communication research as ideological practice. *Communication Theory*, 1(3), 179–203.

Signposting

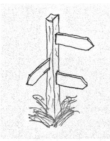

If the ideas in this book have piqued your interest and you would like to find out more about training to become a systemic practitioner at intermediate level or qualify as a systemic and family psychotherapist you will find further information and resources in the training section of the website of the Association for Family Therapy and Systemic Practice in the UK.

www.aft.org.uk

Glossary

Ableism: The oppression that arises from seeing and creating our experience of the world and humanity only through a non-impaired perspective. A certain kind of self or person is held to be normative. Those who do not meet this norm are viewed as a diminished form of the human.

Both/And position: The recognition that frequently things are simultaneously and/or alternately *both* one thing *and* another, e.g. my children have *both* the best mother they have ever had *and* the worst mother they have ever had, all in the same person; living with a learning disability can be *both* a challenge *and* utterly amazing. It invites us to seek multiple descriptions, stories and meanings, to consider multiple contexts and be open to possibilities and reframing.

Circularity: The continuous weaving and reweaving of feedback from a system (responses, thoughts, ideas and language) back into it, creating opportunities for shifts in sense making, thoughts and ideas about what is happening. A professional may facilitate this by asking questions about relationships (see circular questioning).

Circular questioning: A technique for conducting a conversation in a supportive and curious way that invites the participants to triangulate each other's responses in order to gain new ways of making sense of the situation rather than to establish an objective truth – e.g. *What do you suppose she makes of that? Is that how you see it? Did you know that she thought you were thinking that? If I asked him to answer this question what do you suppose he might say?*

Coordinated Management of Meaning (CMM): A communication theory that that has been used by many systemic therapists. For CMM communication is the process by which we make our social worlds. This view is often contrasted with the transmission model of communication in which messages are passed from one (always already formed) person to another. If persons, relationships, institutions and cultures are made, they can be remade.

Cultural genogram: A visual representation of, usually, at least three generations; a family tree incorporating aspects of diversity and intergenerational patterns that may include: learning disability; ethnic origin; abuse; substance misuse; religion; education; and other familial patterns.

Curiosity: A key tenet of Milan-style thinking. When we engage our curiosity we seek to understand the relations between those with whom we meet: how they relate to one another, to ideas and to culture more generally. When we work with curiosity we put our assumptions to one side and seek to understand the assumptions of clients and their networks. As we engage with curiosity we hope to spark curiosity in the minds of everyone.

Dialogical: To be in a dialogue is to be in a conversation where all the participants have a voice, all matter, all may contribute to knowledge and sense making. Everyone is open to change and new understanding. We can contrast this with the taking of a monological position wherein our professional selves, ideas and professionalised knowledge are understood to be not open to change in a conversation with those we support.

Disablism: The oppression experienced by people who live with some form of impairment. It can occur deliberately or unconsciously, e.g. it makes presumptions about quality of life, capacity, or what is possible.

Domains of production, explanation, aesthetics: A systemic tool that helps us to consider the kinds of conversational episodes we are co-creating. The domain of explanation is the domain that is predominantly described in a book such as this. This is the aspect of a conversation where meanings are explored and stories recounted and developed and so on. When we move into the domain of production we privilege the contexts of legalities, professional duties and safety. These concepts draw our attention to the importance of moving between these domains in a way that allows them to coexist in a particular professional relationship; the art of managing these domains is described as the domain of aesthetics.

Epistemology: A theoretical way of knowing, understanding and making sense of something and what is known about it.

First-order change: Change that occurs in a linear fashion, e.g. a target behaviour is reduced or altered. It has been described as a kind of change that does not alter the logic or rules of the relationships and contexts in which it is embedded.

Guide to a Good Day (G2GD): G2GD is a solution-focused tool that follows a traffic light – green, amber, red – structure for increasing the chance of a good day.

Genogram: A visual representation of multiple generations of a family tree, typically using shapes or symbols to represent people.

Homeostasis: The concept that describes a system's tendency to return to a particular state via negative (change-minimising) feedback. This concept was adopted by early systems thinkers, and although it arguably retains explanatory power, later thinkers argued the concept was too mechanistic to usefully describe the complexity and reflexivity of human social systems.

Hypothesising: An idea and/or formulation about what might be happening in relationships in a complex system that may or may not be correct or useful. Ideas are not developed to prove that they are true but rather to explore current thinking and possibilities in the hope of new conversations and sense making together.

Intersectionality: A way of thinking about diversity and oppression that recognises that each person's experience of the multiplicity and interplay of their own aspects of similarity and difference will create a unique pattern of oppression that is influenced by culture and society. For example, consider the ways in which a black British, 'learning disabled' lesbian might experience oppression.

Interventive interviewing: Asking questions concerns far more than seeking information. Asking questions influences the direction work takes and how those to whom the questions are addressed may experience themselves and each other (and the therapist). Asking questions is therefore not a neutral activity. Therapists take responsibility for the questions they ask; for example if they choose to ask about abilities or deficits, diagnoses or friends, comorbidities or dreams of the future. This idea recognises that we cannot ask questions without sharing our own perspective; we could have used another word, asked about a different aspect of the client's experience, asked a different person and so on. These questions always have the potential to create contexts for change. So we need to be thoughtful, curious and aware of what those changes might be.

Irreverence: The ability to know something well enough that you are able to disregard it in favour of alternative beliefs and actions when they are more appropriate.

Learning disability: A socially constructed, legally recognised term that can be sought out by people seeking access to specific resources and allocated by people in powerful positions, and has the potential effect of labelling a person as being 'other' and devalued throughout their lifetime.

LUUUUTT Model: A tool from the Coordinated Management of Meaning approach. This tool enables us to gather a richer picture of a system. LUUUUTT draws attention to the ways in which systems are being described. It prompts us to ask about the stories (meanings/perspectives/events/situations and so on) being lived, untold, unheard, unknown, untellable, told, and the manner of storytelling. We can, for example, ask about what is and what is not being talked about in a person's life (are there stories of blame and shame?), or what a referral to a specialist team tells us and does not, or consider whether, how and with whom a person with learning disabilities' voice is not heard, and where it might be heard and be powerful.

Narrative therapy: An approach to therapy developed by Michael White and David Epston. This approach explores the stories that make up people's lives. At times people and problems can be seen as synonymous: he 'has' an anger problem, they are a 'difficult' family, she 'has' challenging behaviour. For narrative therapy, problems and people are separate. People are not problems; problems are problems. Narrative therapy (see Chapter 4 of this volume) supports people and their networks of relationships to find ways of developing new stories and influence over problems.

Network meeting: An opportunity for everyone involved in a system to come together (for example the person, their family, professionals and key community members), usually around a person with a learning disability, to gain insight and share their expertise, knowledge and resources. As those present engage in a dialogue the relations between those in the meeting (and those who are invoked who are not there) are made visible in the conversations. The facilitator(s) may hold in mind the seeking out of the network's intentions, abilities and strengths. The meeting seeks to improve systemic understanding and co-create ways of supporting the person more effectively.

Neutrality: Taking the position that you are there for everyone in the room and no one in particular at the same time, so that everyone thinks that you are, at least to some extent, on their side.

Open dialogue: An approach originating in primary mental health services. Services respond quickly in crises through meetings with the individual, their family, professionals and social circle to help them make change possible in a collaborative and mutual endeavour – in some ways similar to a rapid and issue-specific circle of support in response to a crisis of some kind (see also network meeting).

Paradox: Something that seems to be nonsensical or contradictory but may actually be well founded. Paradoxes can operate at the levels of meaning, language and action, and in individuals, groups of people (families and staff teams) and organisations. Often paradoxes leave people feeling stuck, but taking time to consider them may offer useful insights and new perspectives.

Positive connotation: A way to make sense of a behaviour or speech act that gives it a positive relational spin. We co-create a positive connotation when we develop new meanings with clients that recognise the good intentions of those who engage in behaviours that may be nevertheless unwanted. In this way we position those in the system as having the possibility of being part of the creation of new, more hopeful ways of relating.

Power: A capacity or ability to control, influence, direct, manage or lead. It can be taken and/or given to you by others; be used overtly or covertly; exist as power to act or power over something, e.g. power is exercised in deciding what is discussed, by whom, how and when.

Prejudice: The recognition that we always have ideas about what we are doing. This suggests it is not possible to be neutral but we can keep a watchful eye on the ideas we are drawing upon, that are influencing us. This use of the word 'prejudice' includes any idea, experience, belief, theory, pattern or story (professional, societal and familial), that influences how we think and act. Some of these ideas will be more or less useful in different circumstances. Reflective practitioners should see themselves as a treasure trove of prejudices. Our task is to get to know what is in our own treasure chest well enough that we are able to be optimally useful, flexible and, at the very least, not detrimental to our own best practice.

Psycho-emotional disablism: The oppression experienced by disabled people that impacts upon their sense of identity, worth and well-being.

Relational: A description of the what and how of people being in relationship together. It can include language, sense making, dialogue, action, non-verbal communication, senses, feelings and visual considerations to name just a few. In systemic practice the relational is foregrounded and persons are formed by relations between people and ideas. To relate differently is to *be* differently.

Relational reflexivity: When two or more people explore how they communicate to investigate and enhance how they are able to work together and make sense of each other. It can be described as 'talking about talking'.

Reflecting team: One or more people who witness a process (discussion, consultation, conversation, supervision, therapeutic session) and offer their thoughts and ideas about what they notice and how they make sense of it in the interests of assisting the outcomes of that process.

Reflective: The ability to consider the what, why and how of something as you are doing it and adjust your actions in the moment to achieve better practice.

Reflexive: Being able to look back on something and learn from it; also considered reflection *on* action.

Reframe: To describe a situation by looking at it in a different way and in such a way that it can change the way the original thing is understood.

Relationship to help: The different ideas that we all have about what help we think we need, are entitled to and can accept that affect both how we *offer* and *receive* assistance from others.

Recursive: Being woven back into and reconsidered over and over.

Safe uncertainty: A way to manage the risks inherent in making change. When we are open to possibilities and able to be less certain of our ideas, change becomes possible. This is most likely when we approach this uncertainty from positions, contexts, language and relationships that are open, warm and secure.

Scripts (family): Repeated, often unconscious, patterns of relating to each other learnt over time. Frequently used in describing families but can be present in staff teams and other groups.

Second-order change: Occurs when there is a change in the way that a problem is understood that makes it seem like a different sort of issue or possibly not an issue at all.

Social Graces (also Social GRRAACCES): A mnemonic that can usefully remind us about, and help us to reflexively attend to, aspects of diversity, sameness and difference. This includes characteristics protected under the Equality Act 2010 among others, namely: gender, geography, race, religion, age, ability, appearance, class, culture, ethnicity, education, employment, sexuality, sexual orientation, spirituality. Social Graces can be both visible/invisible and voiced/unvoiced. The Social Graces concept has been criticised for being limited to certain characteristics and also in potentially drawing our focus away from the intersectional nature of diversity and oppression.

Social model of disability: An approach that considers that disability is brought about by physical barriers (e.g. steps), attitudes and stigma (e.g. 'people with learning disabilities don't do that', hate crime), information (in non-accessible formats) and institutions (e.g. segregated educational provision or benefit restrictions making people wary of seeking a job) that restrict people who live with impairments and may result in disablement.

Systemic: Evolving from theories of cybernetics and considering that meaning is made in language, expectations, duties and relationships, a systemic approach highlights that the interconnected and interdependent nature of the world we live in is composed of a multitude of systems including language, the systems of our physical bodies, the physical world around us and myriad social contexts. These contexts form us and how we make sense of the world.

Systemic formulation: A theory about why something is happening that is not linear and problem focused but rather incorporates connections and meaning-making between everyone in the network or system and considers how their relating to and with each other is making their experience.

Transmission model: An approach to understanding communication sometimes used in comparison to the Coordinated Management of Meaning (CMM) social constructionist approach to communication (sometimes called the communication approach). Where CMM views communication as a process that is informed by and in-forms those in communication creating episodes, selves, relationships, family identities, institutions and the wider cultures we inhabit; the transmission model focuses on information exchange between already formed selves and the processes of coding and decoding messages. The social constructionist approach allows us to consider what our communication 'makes'. For example we can ask: how does this way of talking together influence how a person might understand themselves and how others might understand them, and what possibilities might this open up or constrain?

Warming the context: Talking about talking, and preparing the people engaging in a particular type of conversation for what to expect both before the conversation and moment by moment.

Index